Study Guide to accompany

MOSBY'S
Comprehensive
Dental Assisting

A CLINICAL APPROACH

BETTY LADLEY FINKBEINER, CDA, RDA, BS, MS

Chairperson, Dental Assisting Program
Washtenaw Community College
Ann Arbor, Michigan

CLAUDIA SULLENS JOHNSON, RDA, BS

Clinical Instructor, Dental Assisting Program
Washtenaw Community College
Ann Arbor, Michigan

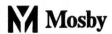 Mosby

St. Louis Baltimore Boston
Carlsbad Chicago Naples New York Philadelphia Portland
London Madrid Mexico City Singapore Sydney Tokyo Toronto Wiesbaden

Executive Editor: Linda L. Duncan
Developmental Editor: Penny Rudolph
Project Manager: Patricia Tannian
Senior Production Editor: Barbara Jeanne Wilson
Senior Book Designer: Gail Morey Hudson
Manufacturing Supervisor: Karen Lewis
Cover Art: Gail Morey Hudson

Printed in the United States of America
Printing/binding by Plus

Mosby-Year Book, Inc.
11830 Westline Industrial Drive
St. Louis, Missouri 63146

94 95 96 97 98 / 9 8 7 6 5 4 3 2 1

PREFACE

This study guide is intended to supplement the textbook *Comprehensive Dental Assisting: A Clinical Approach*. In addition, it may serve as an excellent reference for the person already in the profession who is seeking a review of basic procedures. The following suggestions will help you use this book to identify your strengths and weaknesses, as you seek to evaluate your understanding of various concepts.

Review the contents of each chapter. Before you answer any of the questions or activities, read the printed directions carefully. Review each of the questions thoroughly. When you are responding to multiple-choice questions, keep in mind that you can arrive at the answer in two different ways: first, by *knowing* the answer and finding it among the alternatives offered and, second, by eliminating the incorrect answers, either by knowing that they are wrong or by being able to figure out that they are wrong. Both methods are based on knowing which answers are correct or incorrect. You must arrive at the one correct or *best* answer.

When illustrations or photographs are used in the examination, look at these illustrations thoroughly and identify as many elements as possible; then use the same approach as for the multiple-choice questions—the process of eliminating answers you know are incorrect.

For the lengthier, completion-type questions the authors refer you to the specific chapters to review the possible answers.

Budget your time. Board examinations and many classroom tests are timed. Such examinations are used to simulate actual work experience. Taking a long time at chairside to find an instrument or mix a dental material means a loss in production and ultimately becomes a financial loss for the dentist. Thus, it is common for a dental assistant student to work under time constraints on a test. Quickly look over the number of tasks that are required in a practical examination or the number of questions to be answered in a written examination; then determine the pace at which you will need to work to allow appropriate time to complete each section.

Answer the questions in sequence. Basic concepts are generally presented first, and the more difficult or complex tasks are addressed later. By answering the basic questions first you can build up confidence, which can spur you on to tackle the more difficult problems.

At the end of most chapters are *Clinical Applications* or *Critical-Thinking Activities*, or both. To complete many of these, you will need peer or instructor input. Sometimes, answers will differ in various areas of the country, depending on the state laws. In addition, a puzzle has been provided to lighten up the learning experience and perhaps offer a different type of challenge.

If you are unable to answer a question, leave it and go on to the next area. Sometimes, a person cannot recall a certain concept or procedure. Some tasks or questions may take longer to read and may be more difficult to answer. Therefore, most test takers find it wise to work all the way through an examination at a rapid pace, answering first all the questions they *know* and the questions they can work out the answer to fairly quickly, coming back to some of the more difficult questions later. As you progress to another area in the examination, it is likely that one of the questions or answers may trigger a thought that permits you to successfully return to an unanswered question. It may be that you simply are unable to answer one of the questions. If this occurs, accept it. After you have taken the test, review the material in the textbook that is related to the question that posed difficulty.

When you use the approach of moving through the test fairly rapidly and skipping some questions, you must be particularly cautious in locating accurately the answer space for each question, if an answer sheet is used. Inaccurately spacing your answers on the answer sheet could create a problem that you might not notice until later in the testing; to correct the spacing of your answers is a waste of time.

<u>Check your work</u>. Once all the questions and problems have been answered, refer to the answer section at the back of the study guide to check your work. To refer to this section earlier, denies you the experience of confirming what you really know. Be fair with yourself. When you do well, you can be confident that you have learned the basic concepts and should do well on other similar tests. If you fail in several areas, let the failure serve as impetus to review the material in the textbook or to seek help from an instructor to correct any misunderstanding of the concepts.

CONTENTS

UNIT 1

The Modern Dental Health Team

1 The Modern Dental Health Team

LEARNING OBJECTIVES

You will have mastered the material in this chapter when you can:

- Define the key terms
- Describe the role of each member of the dental health team
- Identify the members of the dental health team
- Describe the background of the dentist and the dental auxiliaries
- Identify and describe each of the dental specialties
- Describe advanced functions
- Identify acronyms common to the dental profession
- Identify the factors or programs that influenced changes in dentistry
- Explain the concept of team dentistry
- Identify the objectives of dentistry

KEY TERMS

Advanced functions
American Dental Association (ADA)
Certified Dental Assistant (CDA)
Certified Dental Technician (CDT)
Certified Orthodontic Assistant (COA)
Certified Dental Practice Management Assistant (CDPMA)
Certified Oral and Maxillofacial Surgery Assistant COMSA
Chairside clinical assistant
Doctor of Dental Surgery (DDS)
Dental assistant
Dental Assistant National Board (DANB)
Dental health team
Dental laboratory technician
Dental practice act
Dental Public Health
Dentist
Dentistry
Doctor of Dental Medicine (DMD)
Endodontics
Etiology
General practitioner

Oral maxillofacial surgery
Oral pathology
Orthodontics
Pediatric dentistry
Periodontics
Prosthetics
Registered Dental Assistant (RDA)
Registered Dental Assistant in Expanded Functions (RDAEF)
Registered Dental Hygienist (RDH)
Specialty
State Board of Dentistry

FILL-IN QUESTIONS

Define the following acronyms.

1. ADA
2. CDA
3. CDT
4. COA
5. CDPMA
6. COMSA
7. DDS
8. DANB
9. RDA
10. RDAEF
11. RDH
12. DMD
13. List the eight recognized specialties of dentistry.

    a. _____

    _____

    b. _____

    _____

    c. _____

    _____

    d. _____

    _____

e. _____

_____

f. _____

_____

g. _____

_____

h. _____

_____

14. In each of the following situations name the specialist to whom a general dentist might refer a patient for treatment.
   a. A person is interested in starting a clinic for children with special needs in a local school district.

   _____

   b. The patient has severe malocclusion.

   _____

   c. The dentist has identified disease within the pulp of a tooth.

   _____

   d. The supporting tissues around a patient's tooth are severely inflamed, and the bone support is in jeopardy.

   _____

   e. A child displays severe emotional problems and needs extensive dental treatment.

   _____

15. List the members of the dental health team.

   _____

   _____

   _____

_____

16. Who is the most important person in the dental office?

_____

17. What is the suffix used to identify the science or study of a specialized area in dentistry?

_____

18. What is the suffix used to identify the person who practices a specialized area of dentistry?

_____

19. List the responsibilities of each member of the dental health team. List the member in the space provided, then give a brief but complete description of the duties.

   MEMBER

   a. _____

   b. _____

   c. _____

   d. _____

   PRIMARY RESPONSIBILITIES

   a. _____

   b. _____

   c. _____

   d. _____

MATCHING QUESTIONS

From the list below choose the one best term that defines each of the following statements.
a. CDT
b. CDA
c. DDS
d. RDH
f. RDAEF

20. ____ A person with a credential granted from the DANB

21. ____ Licensed person whose primary role is preventive treatment

22. ____ Performs extraoral functions, primarily the construction of prosthetic devices

23. ____ Meets the requirements in some states to perform intraoral duties

MULTIPLE-CHOICE QUESTIONS

24. The national professional organization for a dental assistant is the
    a. ADA
    b. ADAA
    c. ADHA
    d. NADA

25. The group responsible for establishing regulations that govern the practice of dentistry within a state is the
    a. American Dental Association
    b. Dental Assistant National Board
    c. Commission on Dental Accreditation
    d. Board of Dentistry

26. Which of the following duties is considered an advanced function for dental assistants in some states?
    a. Scaling teeth
    b. Oral evacuation
    c. Administration of local anesthesia
    d. Placing and carving amalgam restorations

CRITICAL THINKING ACTIVITIES

1. A dental practice is a health care facility, but it is also a business. What factors might be involved in making it a productive business?
2. You enter a new position in a dental practice and are asked to perform certain duties for which you are unsure of the legal requirements. What would you do and to what could you refer to ensure that you are performing duties for which you are legally qualified?

```
V I M N Q G M A L O C C L U S I O N D M N V R X L O
I N L S T U E V R T S I L A I C E P S S P P O A V P
C M A S C I T N O D O H T S O R P E B A A P N N D Q
T L N K J W V Y E T I O L O G Y F R B D T A O D D R
U S O H O N P E O R T H O D O N T I C S C Q D R S Z
P E I E R A C H T L A E H V Q S P O U T T R L A R M
E A E C O E V I T N E V E R P G R N D S A T I B Z I
C I F P A T I E N T T I A S S I S T A N T N C C D H
I L O T E N V Y T O G R E S N E C I L F I A A T N T
T I R O D D S O G Y D R A D N A T S H C E R B V A E
C X P U B L I C H E A L T H D E N T I S T R Y R V N
A U R A B C L A B O R A T O R Y T E C H N I C I A N
R A U P T T D E T S N O I T C N U F D E C N A V D A
P L E D I H R F G R H I J R V I C R E D E N T I A L
M A X I L L O F A C I A L O R A L S U R G E R Y P O
A T H O T P O L A T O C R N V S T R B C E O F N H S
E N P O T N Z F O R E N S I C S U O I N F E A D R R
T E W U X T D I A G N O S I S V O S H A P P R E A A
V D T S E F N I D V Y R S R E G A N A M E D I F F O
```

In the puzzle find the words listed below, which relate to the dental health team. The words are in the puzzle in a horizontal, vertical, or diagonal pattern in two directions.

ADA   ETHICS   DENTAL AUXILIARIES
CDA   STANDARD   HEALTH CARE
RDA   CLINIC   OFFICE MANAGER
RDH   TEETH   ADVANCED FUNCTIONS
DDS   CREDENTIAL   LABORATORY TECHNICIAN
DMD   PATIENT   TEAM PRACTICE
EFDA   DIAGNOSIS   ROOT CANAL
RDAEF   HYGIENIST   MALOCCLUSION
OSHA   ASSISTANT   SPECIALIST
PEDIATRIC   ORTHODONTICS   ENDODONTICS
ETIOLOGY   PROSTHODONTICS   MAXILLOFACIAL ORAL SURGERY
PREVENTIVE   PROFESSIONAL   PERIODONTIST
PATHOLOGY   ROOT CANAL   PUBLIC HEALTH DENTISTRY
GENERAL   LICENSE   FORENSICS
ETIOLOGY   RADIOGRAPH

2   Evolution of the Dental Assistant

LEARNING OBJECTIVES

You will have mastered the material in this chapter when you can:

- Define the key terms
- Describe the role of the modern dental assistant
- Explain the origin of dental assisting
- Describe a brief history of dental assisting
- Define the purpose of the American Dental Assistants' Association
- Describe the evolution of education for the dental assistant
- Identify credentialing processes for dental assistants
- Identify individuals who have made significant contributions to the history of dental assisting
- Explain the impact of DAU on the profession of dental assisting
- Discuss changes that have impacted the dental profession in recent decades
- Explain potential job sources for dental assistants

KEY TERMS

American Association of Dental Schools (AADS)
American Dental Assistants' Association (ADAA)
Commission on Dental Accreditation CDA)
Council on Dental Education (CDE)
Dental Auxiliary Teacher Education (DATE)
Dental Auxiliary Utilization (DAU)
Four-handed dentistry

FILL-IN QUESTIONS

1. List five situations other than working in a general or specialty practice as a clinical chairside assistant or an office manager that a qualified dental assistant might consider for employment.

   a. _____

   b. _____

   c. _____

   d. _____

   e. _____

2. The person credited with hiring the first dental assistant was

   _____.

3. The first state to license dental assistants was

   _____.

MULTIPLE-CHOICE QUESTIONS

4. DAU grants given in the mid-1900s by the federal government to dental schools were used to
   a. Teach dental students to work with dental assistants
   b. Train dental assistants
   c. Train dental students in practice management

5. Which of the following statements are *not* true regarding dental assistant credentialing
   1. Dental assistants are licensed in all states.
   2. Credentials verify professional credibility.
   3. Certification from DANB is a prerequisite to be eligible for state licensure.
   4. General and specialty credentials are offered through the DANB.

   a. 1 and 3
   b. 2 and 4
   c. 1, 2, 3
   d. All of the above

CRITICAL-THINKING ACTIVITIES

1. Consider the program in which you are currently enrolled. What impact does the Commission on Dental Accreditation have on this program? Why is this important to you?

2. You are nearing graduation from a dental assistant program. What types of credentials can you obtain from the school itself? For what types of external credentials are you eligible to apply? What significance will these credentials have for your employment?

UNIT 1I

Basic Sciences in Dentistry

3 Basic Anatomy and Physiology

LEARNING OBJECTIVES

You will have mastered the material in this chapter when you can:

- Define the key terms
- List common prefixes and suffixes relative to dentistry
- Describe anatomic position
- Describe anatomic body locations
- Explain the different body planes
- Explain the human organism and cell components
- Identify the basic systems of the body as they relate to dentistry
- Identify and locate the bones and other important landmarks of the skull
- Identify and locate muscles of mastication and facial expression and the origin and insertion of each
- Identify the oral cavity and facial landmarks
- Identify and list the parts and name the purpose of the temporomandibular joint
- Identify the location and the purpose of the salivary glands and the surrounding structures
- Identify and describe the paranasal sinuses and functions of each

KEY TERMS

Alveolar process
Anatomic position
Anatomy
Anomalies
Anterior
Artery
Atria
Blood
Body planes
Bone
Canal
Cells
Condyle
Cranial bones
Deglutition
Distal

Dorsal
Extrinsic
Facial bones
Foramen
Fossa
Frenum
Frontal
Inferior
Insertion
Intrinsic
Lateral
Longitudinal
Mandible
Maxilla
Meatus
Medial
Mesial
Muscles of Facial Expression
Muscles of Mastication
Neuron
Orbit
Organ
Origin
Osteoblast
Osteoclast
Papilla
Periosteum
Physiology
Posterior
Process
Protuberance
Proximal
Ramus
Sagittal
Salivary glands
Septum
Sinus
Superior
Suture
Symphysis
Synovial
System
Temporomandibular Joint
Tissue
Transverse
Tubercle

Vein
Ventral
Ventricle
Vestibule

FILL-IN QUESTIONS

1. What two functions does the buccinator muscle perform?

   _____

   _____

2. What enzyme does a salivary gland excrete?

   _____

3. Which of the paranasal sinuses has the greatest significance in dentistry? Explain why this is true.
   a. Name of sinus: _____

   b. Reasons for importance: _____

   _____

4. List two functions of the paranasal sinuses:

   _____

   _____

5. What branch of the external carotid artery supplies the teeth?

   _____

6. What nerve innervates the muscles of mastication?

   _____

7. What nerve innervates the muscles of facial expression?

   _____

8. Name the bones that make up the neurocranium.

   _____

   _____

_____

_____

_____

_____

9. Name the bones that make up the viscerocranium.

   _____

   _____

   _____

   _____

   _____

   _____

   _____

10. Name the structures indicated by each line.

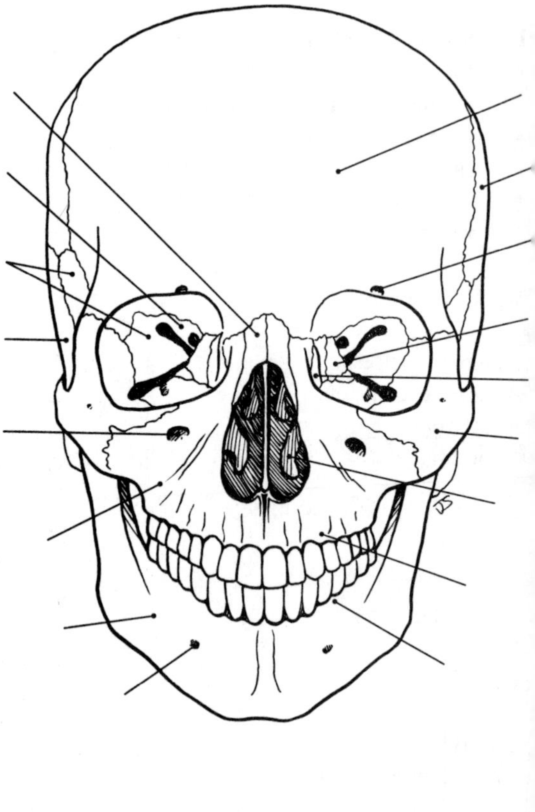

FIG. 3-1 Frontal view of the skull.

11. Name the structures indicated by each line.

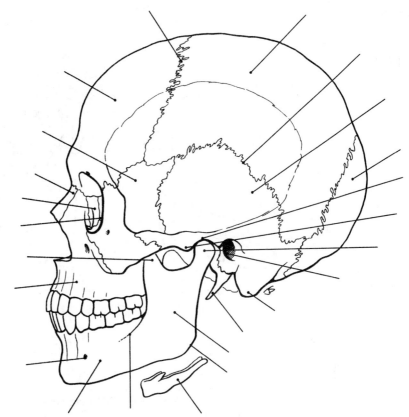

FIG. 3-2 Lateral view of the skull.

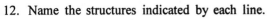

12. Name the structures indicated by each line.

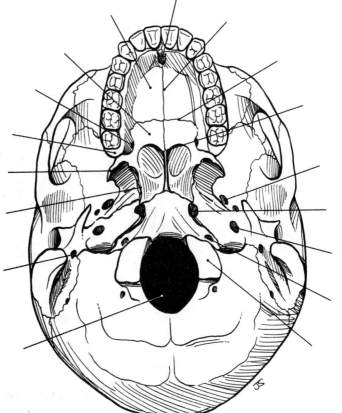

FIG. 3-3 Inferior view of the skull.

13. Name the structures indicated by each line.

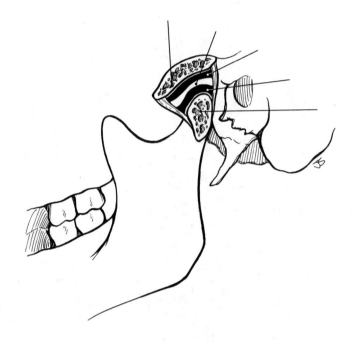

FIG. 3-4 TMJ diagram.

14. Name the structures indicated by each line.

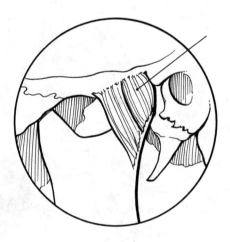

FIG. 3-5 Lateral view of the muscle structure.

5. Name the structures indicated by each line.

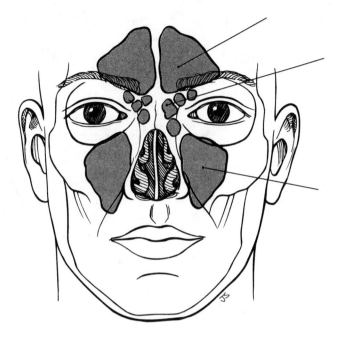

FIG. 3-6 Frontal view of the sinuses.

6. Name the structures indicated by each line.

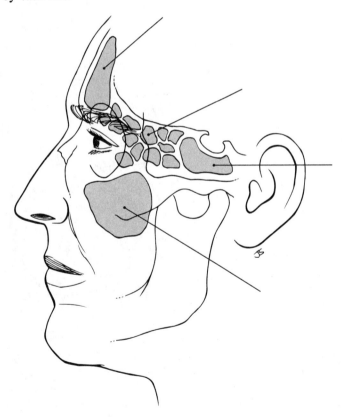

FIG. 3-7 Lateral view of the sinuses.

17. Name the structures indicated by each line.

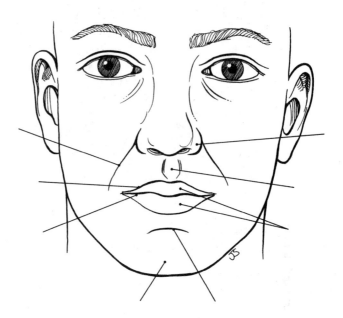

FIG. 3-8 Frontal view of the face.

18. Name the structures indicated by each line.

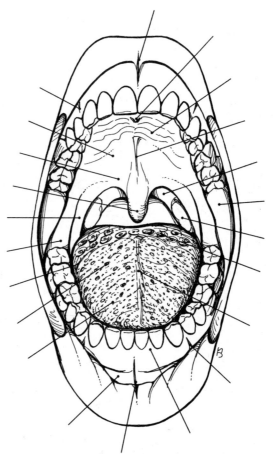

FIG. 3-9 Open mouth.

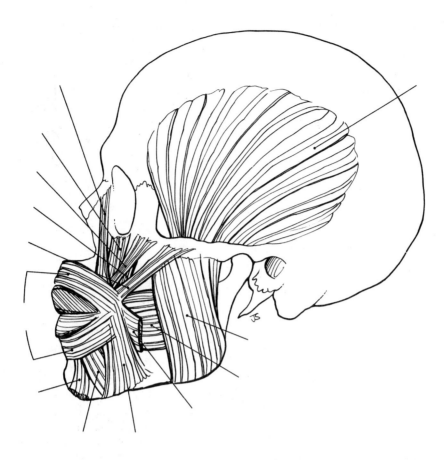

FIG. 3-10 The muscles of mastication and facial expression.

MATCHING QUESTIONS

Match the terms below with the appropriate definitions.

_____ 19. Elevation   a. Raising or closing
_____ 20. Retrusion   mandible
_____ 21. Lateral   b. Moving forward
       excursion   c. Moving back
_____ 22. Protrusion   d. Lowering or opening
                     mouth
                 e. Moving sideways

Match the terms below with the best answer:

a. Lambdoidal   f. Foramen
b. Sagittal   g. Fossa
c. Coronal   h. Ramus
d. Squamosal   i. Septum
e. Condyle

_____ 23. A pit or depression in bone
_____ 24. The suture between the frontal and parietal bones

_____ 25. The suture between the parietal and temporal bones
_____ 26. Vertical portion of the mandible
_____ 27. Tubular, narrow passage through bone
_____ 28. A dividing wall or partition made of a thin plate of bone
_____ 29. The suture between the parietal bones
_____ 30. A hole or perforation in bone

MULTIPLE-CHOICE QUESTIONS

31. The CNS consists of the following:
    1. Brain
    2. Spine
    3. Spinal cord
    4. Parasympathetic system
    5. Sympathetic system

    a. 1 and 3
    b. 2 and 4
    c. 1, 3 and 5
    d. 1, 2, 3 and 4
    e. All of the above

32. The chambers of the heart include the following:
    1. Right and left ventricle
    2. Right and left aorta
    3. Right and left atrium
    4. Right and left jugular
    5. Right and left carotid

    a. 1 and 2
    b. 1 and 3
    c. 2 and 4
    d. 3 only
    e. 4 only

33. When a patient is positioned to be lying on the back with face up, this position is referred to as the following:
    a. Dorsal
    b. Supine
    c. Lateral
    d. Ventral

34. A plane that provides a cross-section of the body is referred to as the following:
    a. Frontal
    b. Horizontal
    c. Sagittal
    d. Longitudinal

TRUE OR FALSE QUESTIONS

Place a **T** for True or an **F** for False in the space provided as it refers to each of the following statements.

_____ 35. The mandible is superior to the maxilla.
_____ 36. A sagittal cut provides a cross-section.
_____ 37. The buccal surface of a tooth is closest to the cheek.
_____ 38. The mesial and distal surfaces of teeth are considered proximal surfaces.
_____ 39. The tongue surface of a tooth may be considered the lingual or palatal surface, depending on the arch in which the tooth rests.
_____ 40. The oral cavity can be divided into six segments and four quadrants.
_____ 41. The incisal surface of teeth refers to the biting surface of all teeth.

CLINICAL APPLICATION

With a patient (classmate) and in a prepared treatment room, identify the following structures on each other:
    a. Inner and outer canthus of the eye
    b. Ala of the nose
    c. Commissure and vermilion border
    d. Synthesis
    e. Vestibule
    f. Alveolar crest
    g. Sublingual caruncle
    h. Uvula
    i. Gingiva
    j. Mucosa
    k. Rugae
    l. Circumvallate papilla
    m. Parotid gland
    n. Soft palate
    o. Interdental papilla
    p. Maxillary tuberosity
    q. Retromolar pad
    r. Median palatine suture
    s. Maxillary frenum
    t. Sublingual frenum
    u. Buccal mucosa
    v. Dorsal surface of the tongue
    w. Inferior surface of the ear
    x. Lateral area of the eye
    y. Temporal bone
    z. Occipital bone

CRITICAL-THINKING ACTIVITIES

1. Reflect on the various systems of the body, and explain how each relates to the various facets of dentistry, such as development of oral tissues and dental treatment.

2. A patient contacts the dental office and indicates that his or her teeth "hurt" toward the posterior of the mouth. Recently the patient had a cold, and now it hurts when he or she closes the teeth together. What might these symptoms indicate?

4 Intraoral Structures

LEARNING OBJECTIVES

You will have mastered the material in this chapter when you can:

- Define the key terms
- Identify each dentition
- List the teeth and the characteristics of each dentition
- Locate the dentition, arch, and quadrant of each dentition
- Describe common tooth numbering systems as they correlate to specific teeth.
- Describe oral histology and embryology and their relationship to the oral cavity
- Describe the functions of the teeth and surrounding tissues
- Explain the difference between the anatomic and clinical crown
- List and identify the parts of the tooth
- Describe the development of the tooth from bud stage through eruption
- List the sequence of eruption of both dentitions

KEY TERMS

Ameloblast
Angle
Apical foramen
Attrition
Axial
Bell stage
Buccal
Bud
Canine
Cap stage
Cementoblast
Cementum
Cingulum
Concave
Contact
Convex
Crown
Curve of Spee
Cusp
Cuspid

Deciduous
Dentin
Dentinal tubule
Dentition
Diastema
Ectoderm
Embrasure
Embryology
Enamel
Enamel cuticle
Endoderm
Facial
Fibroblast
Fossa
Furcation
Gingiva
Groove
Incisal
Incisor
Histology
Labial
Lamina dura
Lingual
Lobe
Mamelon
Mandible
Maxilla
Mesoderm
Molar
Mucosa
Oblique
Occlusal
Occlusion
Odontoblasts
Overbite
Overjet
Papilla
Periodontium
Permanent
Premolar
Primary
Primordium
Proximal
Pulp
Quadrant
Ridge

Secondary
Segment
Succedaneous
Sulcus
Supernumerary
Tubercle

FILL-IN QUESTIONS

1. How many teeth are in the permanent dentition?

   _____

2. How many teeth are in the primary dentition?

   _____

3. List the teeth in the quadrant of the permanent dentition

   _____

   _____

   _____

Using the information provided below, complete the following chart by indicating in the blank spaces the tooth number for each of the teeth within each system.

Universal (ADA)	Palmer	FDI
4. 32	_____	_____
5. _____	6⌉	_____
6. 24	_____	_____
7. _____	_____	44
8. T	_____	_____
9. _____	A⌋	_____
10 _____	_____	82

11. If a tooth is numbered 30 in the universal numbering system, what is the same tooth numbered in the opposite quadrant of the same arch? _____ What is this same tooth (#30) numbered if it is on the same quadrant in the opposite arch? _____

12. List the cell responsible for the formation of each of the following:

    a. Enamel _____

    b. Periodontal ligament _____

    c. Cementum _____

    d. Dentin _____

13. List the parts of the dental organ, and describe the function of each:

Part	Function
_____	_____
_____	_____
_____	_____

14. At what age do each of the following teeth normally erupt?

    a. Permanent first molars _____
    b. All the primary dentition _____
    c. Permanent maxillary incisors _____
    d. Third molars _____

15. Name the structures indicated by each line.

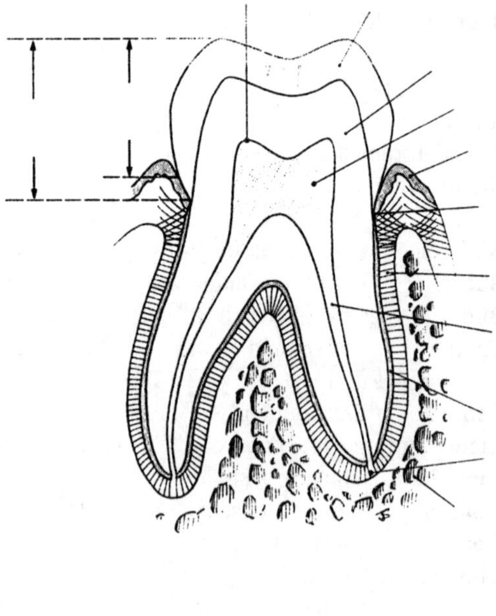

FIG. 4-1 Diagram of tooth.

16. Name the structures indicated by each line. Be specific.

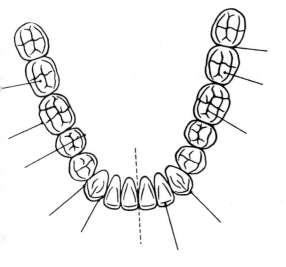

FIG. 4-2 Diagram of the permanent dentition.

MATCHING QUESTIONS

From the list of terms select the brief description that best defines the term.

    a. Pulp canal
    b. Enamel
    c. Dentin
    d. Periodontal fiber
    e. Cementum

17. _____ Hardest tissue in the human body
18. _____ Forms the main portion of the tooth
19. _____ Covers the root
20. _____ Softer than enamel; harder than cementum
21. _____ Protects and supports the tooth but is independent of the tooth's main nourishment system
22. _____ The soft tissue of the tooth
23. _____ Nonliving tissue
24. _____ The union with this tissue and the dentin forms the DEJ
25. _____ The union with this tissue and the enamel forms the CEJ

Match the following conditions with a description:
a. Crossbite
b. Overjet
c. Openbite
d. Overbite
e. Normal bite
f. Edge to edge

26. _____ An existing space between the maxillary and mandibular teeth
27. _____ Facially positioned mandibular teeth
28. _____ Lingually positioned mandibular teeth
29. _____ Deep or vertical overlap of the maxillary teeth on the mandibular teeth beyond what is considered normal edge
30. _____ Contact of the incisal edges rather than interdigitation
31. _____ Horizontal overlap creating protrusion between the labial surface of the mandibular incisors and the lingual surface of the maxillary incisors

MULTIPLE-CHOICE QUESTIONS

32. Which of the following statements are true in relation to the development of the permanent incisors?
    1. They develop apically from the primary incisors
    2. They develop inferior from the primary incisors
    3. Commonly erupt lingually to the primary incisors
    4. Commonly erupt labially to the primary incisors

    a. 1 and 3
    b. 2 and 4
    c. 1, 2, and 3
    d. 4 only

33. The portion of the tooth that is visible above the gingival line is defined as the
    a. Root
    b. Clinical crown
    c. Anatomical crown
    d. Neck of the tooth

34. The area in which a tooth is positioned is called the
    a. Bifurcation
    b. Alveolus
    c. Sulcus
    d. Lamina dura

35. Which of the following teeth generally have two roots?
    a. Permanent maxillary first molars
    b. Permanent mandibular first molars
    c. Permanent maxillary second premolars
    d. Permanent maxillary central incisors

36. The maxillary tooth with the longest root is the
    a. Lateral incisor
    b. Central incisor
    c. Canine
    d. Second molar

37. The largest portion of the pulp that is found in the coronal portion of the tooth is the
    a. Pulp chamber
    b. Pulp canal
    c. Pulp horn
    d. Apical foramen

38. Which of the following teeth are not succedaneous?
    a. Permanent central incisors
    b. Permanent canines
    c. Permanent first molars
    d. Permanent premolars

39. An embrasure is
    a. Usually located toward the cervical aspect of the teeth
    b. The small spot on the mesial or distal surface of teeth at the point of contact
    c. The curvature toward or away from the contact area

40. A ridge extending from the tip of a cusp to the central groove is a(n)
    a. Oblique ridge
    b. Secondary ridge
    c. Transverse ridge
    d. Triangular ridge

41. Rounded elevations of enamel found on the incisal edges of anterior teeth at the time of eruption are known as
    a. Lobes
    b. Cusps
    c. Enamel pearls
    d. Mamelons

42. The roots of the maxillary second molars are the
    a. Mesiolingual, distolingual, and buccal
    b. Mesiobuccal, distobuccal, and palatal
    c. Mesial, distal, and lingual
    d. Mesiolingual, mesiobuccal, and distal

5 Nutrition and Dental Health

LEARNING OBJECTIVES

You will have mastered the material in this chapter when you can:

- Define the key terms
- Explain the difference between the USRDA and RDA
- Explain the food guide pyramid
- Explain energy balance and how it relates to weight gain and loss
- List the major function, food sources, and calories provided per gram for carbohydrates, fats, and proteins.
- List water-soluble vitamins, their function, and food sources
- List fat soluble vitamins, their function, and food sources
- Distinguish between major and trace minerals, and identify their function and food sources
- Explain how to read a food label
- Describe the food exchange system
- Discuss the positive and negative aspects of "fast food" consumption
- Discuss the relationship of monosaccharides, disaccharides, and polysaccharides in caries production
- Identify health risks related to diet
- Explain the effect of medicine and drugs on nutrition
- Discuss dietary management of patients with special needs

KEY TERMS

Calorie
Carbohydrate
Disaccharide
Fat
Fat soluble
Fructose
Galactose
Glucose
kcalorie
Metabolize
Mineral
Monosaccharide
Nutrient
Polysaccharide
Protein
Saccharin
Sucrose
Vitamin
Water soluble

FILL-IN QUESTIONS

1. Differentiate between an unsaturated, a saturated, and a polyunsaturated fatty acid, and give an example of each.

   Type of fatty acid   Example

   _____

   _____

   _____

   _____

2. Provide the function and the results of a deficiency in each of the following fat-soluble vitamins.

Vitamin

   A

   D

   E

   K

Functions

   A

   D

   E

K

Results of deficiency

A

D

E

K

3. Is each of the following minerals considered a major or minor (trace) mineral?

    a. Calcium_____   g. Iron_____

    b. Phosphorus____   h. Iodine_____

    c. Sodium_____   i. Copper_____

    d. Potassium_____   j. Magnesium_____

    e. Chloride_____   k. Fluorine_____

    f. Sulfur_____   l. Zinc_____

4. List five qualities of a dental health care provider when he or she is interviewing a patient during nutritional counseling.

    _____

    _____

    _____

    _____

    _____

5. A. Describe various levels of the Food Pyramid.

    _____

    _____

    _____

    _____

    _____

B. Relate the importance of the Food Pyramid to nutritional health.

    _____

    _____

6. A sample diet obtained from a patient being seen for nutritional counseling includes the following

Breakfast	**Lunch**
8 ounces of grapefruit juice	12 ounce coke
2 cups of coffee	Hot dog with
2 slices of rye toast	sweet relish
w/margarine	Potato salad
1 egg	3 tomato slices

Dinner
8-ounce pork steak
1 cup of asparagus tips
1 small baked potato (dry)
Small tossed salad with vinagarette dressing
1 cup of fresh strawberries

The patient appears to have a relatively healthy diet but has had several carious lesions lately. Some suggestions may be made for dietary improvement. Considering the suggestions provided in the Food Pyramid and its relation to dental disease, what recommendations could be made?

    _____

    _____

    _____

7. What would be a good noncariogenic substitute in the lunch menu of this patient?

    _____

MULTIPLE-CHOICE QUESTIONS

8. The primary function of protein is to:
    a. Contribute to energy metabolism
    b. Play a significant role in the body's resistance to disease
    c. Supply amino acids for building other essential protein substances
    d. Aid the growth and maintenance of tissue

9. A deficiency of vitamin C may result in
    1. Hemorrhagic disease in newborns
    2. Cheilosis
    3. Anemia
    4. Scurvy
    5. Weakness of blood vessels

    a. 1, 4, and 5
    b. 2, 3, and 5
    c. 4 and 5
    d. All of the above

10. Standards for the enrichment of foods is governed by what agency?
    a. Federal Trade Commission
    b. American Dental Association
    c. American Dietary Association
    d. Food and Drug Administration
    e. National Food and Drug Administration

11. Vitamin K can cause
    a. Blood clotting
    b. Cheilosis
    c. Beriberi
    d. Anemia

12. A riboflavin deficiency results in
    a. Malformation of dentinal tubules
    b. Caries prone teenage years
    c. Cheilitis
    d. Herpetic lesion

13. Metabolism is
    a. A steady heart beat
    b. The changes in nutrients by the body
    c. A combination of vascular changes
    d. A respiratory difficulty

14. The following are considered simple sugars
    a. Maltose and glucose
    b. Sucrose and cellulose
    c. Lactose and galactose
    d. Levulose and dextrose

15. Which of the following is known as table sugar?
    a. Sucrose
    b. Maltose
    c. Fructose
    d. Lactose

CLINICAL APPLICATION

The dentist has suggested to the patient that he or she should increase Vitamin C intake. The patient asks you what foods should be eaten to obtain this vitamin. What would you suggest?

CRITICAL-THINKING ACTIVITIES

1. A widowed older adult patient is living by himself in his own home. What intraoral and extraoral evidence might be present to indicate that the patient is malnourished?

2. A young child is seen in the dental office for treatment. The child's appearance seems somewhat different from normal in that there are large shadows under her eyes. What might this symptom indicate?

6   Diseases of the Teeth and Supporting Tissues

LEARNING OBJECTIVES

You will have mastered the material in this chapter when you can:

- Define the key terms
- Recognize normal periodontal tissues
- Recognize the basic signs of periodontal disease
- Differentiate between healthy and unhealthy gingival tissue.
- Describe the progression of periodontal disease, its etiology, and treatment
- Classify the diseases and conditions affecting the calcified portions of the teeth
- Explain the developmental processes of diseases and conditions affecting the calcified portions of the teeth
- Explain the G. V. Black cavity classification
- Describe the classification of cavity forms
- Distinguish between cavity walls, floors and angles used in cavity preparation

KEY TERMS

Abrasion
Acute herpetic gingivostomatitis
Acute Necrotizing Ulcerative Gingivitis (ANUG)
Acute periodontal abscess
Acquired pellicle
Attrition
Calculus
Caries
Cavity preparation
Cavity wall
Convenience form
Erosion
Extrinsic stain
Floor
Gingivitis
Inflammation
Intrinsic stain
Line angle
Materia Alba
Nursing bottle mouth
Outline form
Pericoronitis
Periodontitis
Point angle
Recurrent decay
Reparative dentin
Resistance form
Resorption
Retention form

FILL-IN QUESTIONS

1. Identify the following terms:

   Unilateral cleft:

   Bilateral cleft:

   Cleft lip:

   Cleft palate:

2. Explain the psychologic impact of a cleft palate in a newborn on its mother and family contact persons. How does the cleft palate affect the child as she or he grows older?

MULTIPLE CHOICE QUESTIONS

3. The grinding of teeth is known as
   a. Abrasion
   b. Bruxism
   c. Erosion
   d. Granulation

4. Tetracycline stain is an example of
   a. Intrinsic stain
   b. Extrinsic stain
   c. Fever

5. A cavity preparation that involves two proximal walls and the occlusal surface is _____ and is most likely found on _____.
   1. Class II
   2. Class III
   3. Class IV
   4. Class VI
   5. Anterior teeth
   6. Posterior teeth

   a. 1 and 5
   b. 1 and 6
   c. 2,3, and 5
   d. 2,3, and 6
   e. 4 and 6

6. A cavity preparation that involves one proximal wall and the occlusal surface is _____ and is most likely found on _____.
   1. Class II
   2. Class III
   3. Class IV
   4. Class VI
   5. Anterior teeth
   6. Posterior teeth

   a. 1 and 5
   b. 1 and 6
   c. 2 and 6
   d. 2,3, and 5
   e. 2,3, and 6

7. A cavity preparation that is found on the cervical ⅓ of a posterior tooth is considered a cavity preparation of which class?
   a. Class I
   b. Class II
   c. Class V
   d. Class IV

8. Acute necrotizing ulcerative gingivitis is commonly known as
   a. Epulis
   b. Pregnancy gingivitis
   c. Vincent's disease
   d. Juvenile periodontitis

9. The physiologic wearing away of tooth structure is known as
   a. Atrophy
   b. Attrition
   c. Abrasion
   d. Erosion

10. Green stains found on children's teeth are often the result of
    a. Fluorosis
    b. Tetracycline
    c. Poor oral hygiene
    d. Pyrexia

11. If a stain can be removed with coronal polishing, it is considered to be
    a. Heavy plaque and food
    b. Intrinsic
    c. Extrinsic
    d. Exogenous

12. If teeth appear to have shorter-than-normal roots on a radiograph, the appearance is a result of
    a. Attrition
    b. Abrasion
    c. Normal growth for the individual
    d. Resorption

13. In a mouth that is free of periodontal disease the attached gingiva would appear to be
    a. Boggy
    b. Stippled
    c. Blunted
    d. Smooth

TRUE OR FALSE QUESTIONS

The following statements are True (T) or False (F). Place the correct letter in the space provided for each.

_____ 14. Calculus is usually removed during polishing.
_____ 15. A point angle is where three surfaces meet.
_____ 16. A line angle is where three surfaces meet.
_____ 17. A Class III cavity preparation is located only in anterior teeth.
_____ 18. A Class II cavity preparation is located only in posterior teeth.
_____ 19. Hairy leukoplakia in a patient is pathognomonic for periodontal disease.

_____ 20. Something that is erythematous is usually ulcerated.

_____ 21. Antibiotics are useful for treating oral infections.

CRITICAL-THINKING ACTIVITY

A patient seen in your office needs treatment that will result in Class II and Class VI restorations on two different teeth. The patient is confused and asks about the difference. How would you explain the difference and the reason for this difference?

7   Oral Pathology

LEARNING OBJECTIVES

You will have mastered the material in this chapter when you can:

- Define the key terms
- Identify clinical features, etiology, and treatment information for all conditions
- List the four signs of inflammation
- Identify historical information that should be gathered when lesions are suspected
- Identify the relationship between foliate papillae and the lingual tonsil
- List a differentiating feature between torus mandibularis and exostoses
- Identify oral hygiene information that is appropriate for the patient with a fissured tongue and a hairy tongue
- Identify the time schedule to repair the cleft lip and cleft palate
- Identify the area of the mouth where filiform papillae would be located and the conditions with which they are associated
- Differentiate between characteristics of herpes simplex ulcers and aphthous ulcers
- List features of the four forms of herpetic ulcerations
- Identify precipitating factors for recurrent aphthous ulcers and herpetic ulcers
- Identify the relationship between desquamative gingivitis and lichen planus
- Discuss the rationale for biopsy of leukoplakia and erythroplakia and identify the more dangerous of the two lesions
- Identify the role of early detection when squamous cell carcinoma is present in the mouth
- Compare the similarities and differences between basal cell and squamous cell carcinoma and between carcinoma-in-situ and squamous cell carcinoma
- List conditions that form as a result of frequent irritation
- Describe the differences between hyperplasia and hypertrophy
- Identify the conditions associated with *Candida albicans*

- List drugs reported on the medical history that may manifest orally as gingival hyperplasia
- Discuss the role of opportunistic infection in AIDS
- Identify infection control procedures that prevent the transmission of infectious diseases to dental personnel
- List conditions that can only be identified by radiographs

KEY TERMS

Atrophy
Benign
Bilateral
Biopsy
Carcinoma-in-situ
Clinical description
Congenital
Dysplastic
Erythematous
Etiology
Exophytic
Genetic
Hyperkeratinization
Hyperplasia
Hypertrophy
Idiopathic
Inflammation
Innocuous
Lesion
Leukoplakia
Localized
Malignant
Metastasis
Neoplasm
Nodule
Obturator
Odontogenic
Opportunistic
Palpation
Pathology
Tumor
Unilateral

FILL-IN QUESTIONS

1. What are the cardinal signs of inflammation?

   _____

   _____

   _____

   _____

2. What are examples of injurious agents that may cause pathologic changes in tissues?

   _____

   _____

   _____

   _____

3. A neoplasm refers to the following:

   _____

4. When a lesion is examined what three routine steps should be followed?

   _____

   _____

   _____

5. Explain the following terms.

   Unilateral cleft:

   Bilateral cleft:

   Cleft lip:

   Cleft palate:

6. List four common areas (A to D) where oral cancers occur, and indicate the most common area (E) in which oral cancer may be found.

   a.

   b.

   c.

   d.

   e.

7. Name two common oral complications of radiation exposure.
   a.

   b.

8. Using the chart on the next page, identify lesions in each of the various categories; describe their clinical appearance, etiology, and treatment.

Clinical Appearance	Etiology	Treatment

Developmental Conditions

a.

b.

c.

d.

e.

Diseases of the Mucous Membranes

a.

b.

c.

d.

e.

f.

g.

h.

i.

j.

Malignant and Premalignant Lesions

a.

b.

c.

d.

Hyperplastic Lesions

a.

b.

c.

d.

e.

f.

Aids-Related Lesions

a.

b.

c.

d.

Miscellaneous Conditions

a.

b.

c.

d.

MATCHING QUESTIONS

Match the following terms with the definitions

_____ 9. Bilateral

_____ 10. Dysplastic

_____ 11. Idiopathic

_____ 12. Lesion

_____ 13. Congenital

_____ 14. Unilateral

_____ 15. Atrophy

_____ 16. Benign

_____ 17. Carcinoma

_____ 18. Opportunistic

_____ 19. Sarcoma

a. Condition without clear pathogenesis
b. Infection that occurs because of the ability afforded by the state of the host
c. Decrease in size of an object
d. Not recurrent or progressive
e. Affecting two sides
f. Abnormally developed tissue
g. Malignant tumor in epithelial tissue
h. Affecting one side
i. Pathologically altered tissue
j. Able to produce erosion
k. Malignant tumor of the connective tissue
l. Substance that interacts with an antigen
m. Present at birth

MULTIPLE-CHOICE QUESTIONS

20. A causative factor in a disease or condition may be termed
    a. Pathologic manifestation
    b. Etiologic agent
    c. Symptom
    d. None of the above

21. The study of disease processes, the causes, manifestations, and effects of disease on a living organism, and the alterations in structure resulting from the disease is
    a. Histology
    b. Etiology
    c. Pathology
    d. Microscopic anatomy

22. Small ulcers with necrotic centers and areas of inflammation surrounding them may be found in the oral cavity. These areas are known by the lay person as
    a. Herpes simplex
    b. Lichen planus
    c. Gum boils
    d. Canker sores

23. A condition in which the tongue is characterized by nonuniform pattern of smooth areas resulting from a loss of the epithelium is
    a. Black hairy tongue
    b. Aphthous ulcers
    c. Herpes simplex
    d. Geographic tongue

24. An inflammation of the parotid glands is
    a. Measles
    b. Salivary duct calculi
    c. Mumps
    d. Tetanus

25. A patient complains of bleeding and painful gingiva and a foul odor in the mouth. Evidence of poor oral hygiene indicates that this condition is probably
    a. Periodontal disease
    b. Acute necrotizing ulcerative gingivitis
    c. Leukoplakia
    d. Geographic tongue

26. A cleft lip is caused by a lack of fusions between the
    a. Soft palate and hard palate
    b. Maxillary process
    c. Maxillary process and median nasal process
    d. Frontonasal process and median nasal process

27. An antibody is
    a. An autoimmune disease
    b. An enzyme
    c. Part of the body's defense system
    d. None of the above

28. The spreading of cancer to various sites in the body is known as
    a. Toxemia
    b. Carcinoma
    c. Metastasis
    d. Articulation

29. A patient with a history of convulsive seizures has been treated with Dilantin for the past 3 years. A resultant condition that may be manifested in the oral cavity is
    a. Rampant dental caries
    b. Squamous cell carcinoma
    c. Enamel hypoplasia
    d. Gingival hyperplasia

30. An older adult male patient has evidence of a hard bony growth in the palate. This area will have to be removed before placement of an upper denture. The condition is known as a
    a. Torus mandibularis
    b. Toris palatinus
    c. Papilloma
    d. Epulis

31. Koplik's spots are associated with which of the following system diseases?
    a. Leukemia
    b. Diabetes
    c. Measles
    d. Pernicious anemia

32. The clinical symptoms of lichen planus resemble which of the following conditions?
    a. Leukoplakia
    b. Geographic tongue
    c. Dental fluorosis
    d. Squamous cell carcinoma

33. Mulberry molars are an example of
    a. Enamel hypoplasia
    b. Hereditary opalescent dentin
    c. Anodontia
    d. Enamel hyperplasia

34. Which of the following is an example of a sarcoma?
    a. Torus
    b. Papilloma
    c. Fibroma
    d. None of the above

35. Oral conditions that are commonly seen in a patient with AIDS include
    1. Mucocele
    2. Kaposi's sarcoma
    3. Fordyce granules
    4. Hairy leukoplakia

    a. 1 and 3
    b. 2 and 4
    c. 1, 2, and 3
    d. 4 only

36. The following is an oral fungal infection:
    a. Thrush
    b. Herpes
    c. A melanoma
    d. Aphthous ulcer

CLINICAL APPLICATION

Using universal precautions in a treatment room, examine the mouth of a peer for normal and nonnormal conditions of the oral cavity.

CRITICAL-THINKING ACTIVITIES

1. A patient who is in the treatment room shows you a lesion in the mouth. You have an understanding of oral lesions. The patient asks you what you think the oral lesion is. What is your response?

2. A similar situation arises at a social event when a friend or relative asks you a similar question. What is your response in this situation?

8   Infection Control

LEARNING OBJECTIVES

You will have mastered the material in this chapter when you can:

- Define the key terms
- Describe the methods of infection transmission
- Describe HIV, AIDS, HBV, and other infectious diseases
- Explain infection control
- Explain cross-contamination
- Identify the agencies regulating the dental profession
- Explain the techniques employed to eliminate transmission of infectious diseases
- Describe task categorization
- Describe universal precautions
- Explain the OSHA hazard communication program
- Explain common disinfection and sterilization procedures

KEY TERMS

Acquired Immunodeficiency syndrome (AIDS)
Antimicrobial
Antiseptic
Autogenous
Asepsis
Aseptic technique
Bioburden
Blood borne pathogens
Centers for Disease Control and Prevention (CDC)
Cold disinfection
Contamination
Cross-infection
Direct contact
Disinfection
Environmental Protection Agency (EPA)
Hepatitis B virus (HBV)
Human immunodeficiency virus (HIV)
Immunization
Indirect contact
Infection control
Inhalation
Material Safety Data Sheet (MSDS)
Occupational Safety and Health Administration (OSHA)
Polynitral Gloves
Sanitization
Sterilization
Tuberculosis
Universal precautions

FILL-IN QUESTIONS

1. Identify five transferable diseases that a person might encounter in the dental office.

   _____

   _____

   _____

   _____

2. List five categories of patients with a greater than average chance of harboring HBV.

   _____

   _____

   _____

   _____

   _____

3. Describe the three categories of classification of tasks for dental personnel as outlined by OSHA standards.
   Category I: _____

   _____

   _____

Category II: _____

_____

_____

Category III: _____

_____

_____

4. What is meant by the term *universal precautions*?

_____

_____

5. Identify at least three diseases against which all dental personnel should be immunized.

_____

_____

_____

6. Identify the information in the space provided as it relates to time, temperature, and pressure for each of the following procedures:

Procedure

Steam under
  pressure
Dry heat
Chemical vapor

Time

Steam under
  pressure
Dry heat
Chemical vapor

Temperature

Steam under
  pressure
Dry heat
Chemical vapor

Pressure

Steam under
  pressure
Dry heat
Chemical vapor

Identify the following acronyms.

7. OSHA

8. DHCW

9. AIDS

10. CDC

11. EPA

12. HBV

13. HIV

Explain what each of the following terms means. Use complete sentences, and be thorough in your description.

14. Barrier techniques:

15. Medical waste:

16. Poster 2203:

17. Microbiology:

18. Rank the following conditions in order of greatest exposure to the DHCW

    1. Most common
    2. Less common
    3. Rare

    _____ a. Infectious disease
    _____ b. Contamination
    _____ c. Infection

Describe the following terms as they relate to disease transmission in the dental office. Include in your discussion an example of how each form of transmission might occur in a dental office.

19. Direct transmission

20. Indirect transmission

21. Aerosolization

MATCHING QUESTIONS

Using the list of sterilization/disinfection techniques, which process would be the best method for each of the following situations?

a. Dry heat
b. Steam under pressure
c. Glass bead
d. Cold chemical/immersion disinfection
e. Unsaturated chemical vapor

_____ 22. Requires a protective emulsion on sharp-hinged instruments before use.
_____ 23. Efficient method of sterilization at chairside for small endodontic instruments
_____ 24. A method of destroying some organisms on instruments that cannot be sterilized in a heat source
_____ 25. For the short period of its use, good ventilation is recommended
_____ 26. Does not require a protective emulsion but is capable of sterilization when processed for an hour at the appropriate temperature
_____ 27. To sterilize, the exposure time is 15 to 20 minutes at 20 lb of pressure and at 250° to 260° of temperature
_____ 28. To sterilize, in the omniclave, a special door is attached, and temperature is 300° to 320° for 1 hour
_____ 29. Requires that instruments be thoroughly dried before exposure

From the list below select the best procedure for caring for each of the following contaminated devices or materials.

a. Amalgam waste container
b. Steam under pressure
c. Sharps container
d. Spray/wipe/spray/wipe with surface disinfection
e. Discard
f. Dry heat
g. Cold chemical/immersion
h. Discard in infectious waste container

_____ 30. Explorer
_____ 31. Mouth mirror
_____ 32. Scissors
_____ 33. Handpiece
_____ 34. Saliva ejector
_____ 35. Needle
_____ 36. Amalgam scraps
_____ 37. Cotton rolls from HIV patient
_____ 38. Medicaments
_____ 39. Protective glasses
_____ 40. Plastic chair cover
_____ 41. Cotton pellets
_____ 42. Contra angle
_____ 43. Prophylaxis angle
_____ 44. Glass dappen dish
_____ 45. Scalpel blade
_____ 46. Unused cotton tip applicator
_____ 47. Amalgamator

MULTIPLE-CHOICE QUESTIONS

48. The most common routes of transmission of disease is (are)
    1. Blood
    2. Saliva
    3. Aerosols
    4. Splatter
    5. Kissing

    a. 1, 2, and 3
    b. 1, 2, 3, and 4
    c. 1 only
    d. 1, 2, 3, 4, and 5

49. Barrier coverings may be placed
    1. Before a patient is seated
    2. On light handles
    3. On A/W syringe
    4. On HVE hose
    5. At the end of the day
    6. Only when treating a high-risk patient

    a. 1, 2, and 3
    b. 1, 2, 3, and 4
    c. 2, 3, 4, and 5
    d. 2, 3, 4, and 6

50. If done in accordance with the OSHA guidelines, swabbing a dental unit, operating light, and cabinetry with gauze soaked in a surface disinfectant may be considered a
    a. Cleaning procedure
    b. Disinfectant procedure
    c. Sterilization procedure
    d. Cleaning and disinfectant procedure

51. The physical removal of debris and organisms from the surface of an object is a
    a. Disinfectant procedure
    b. Cleaning procedure
    c. Sterilization procedure
    d. None of the above

52. Which of the following would be the most ideal barrier techniques to protect the dental team?
    1. Use of only sterile instruments
    2. Patient rinse with mouthwash
    3. Complete patient history
    4. Use of HVE
    5. Use of rubber dam

    a. 1 and 3
    b. 2 and 4
    c. 1, 2, 3, and 4
    d. 1, 3, 4, and 5
    e. 1, 2, 3, 4, and 5

53. A health questionnaire completed by a patient indicates that the patient is HIV positive. The DHCW should
    a. Refuse to treat the patient and refer him or her to a local dentist who treats patients with HIV.
    b. Treat the patient as any other patient would be treated.
    c. Delay treatment until the patient recovers.
    d. Tell the patient that the staff does not feel comfortable treating him or her.
    e. Refer the patient to a dentist who has HIV.

54. A health questionnaire completed by a patient indicates that the patient is HBV positive. The DHCW should do the following:
    a. Refuse to treat the patient and refer him or her to a local dentist who treats patients with HBV.
    b. Treat the patient as any other patient would be treated.
    c. Delay treatment until the patient recovers.
    d. Tell the patient that the staff does not feel comfortable treating him or her.
    e. Refer the patient to a dentist who has HIV.

55. A health questionnaire completed by a patient indicates that the patient has tuberculosis. The DHCW should do the following:
    a. Delay treatment until the antibiotic regimen is underway.
    b. Treat the patient as any other patient would be treated.
    c. Refer the patient to a dentist who has tuberculosis.

TRUE OR FALSE

Place a **T** for True or a **F** for False in the space provided as it refers to each of the following statements.

_____ 56. Eating in the sterilization area is permitted providing it is not in the area where instruments are processed.

_____ 57. The general-purpose solution used in an ultrasonic cleaner disinfects as well as cleans the instruments.

_____ 58. An omniclave provides steam under pressure, whereas an autoclave provides the same process, in addition to dry-heat sterilization.

_____ 59. The use of autoclave heat-sensitive tape on a package is proof that the package is sterile.

_____ 60. If a disinfecting immersion instrument solution has a 28-day re-use life, it is always used for 28 days.

_____ 61. Instruments are placed in protective emulsion for 3 to 5 minutes.

_____ 62. A monitoring sterilization system is mandated for use in a dental setting.

_____ 63. Exposure and infection are synonymous terms.

_____ 64. The practice of universal precautions protects only the patient.

_____ 65. All DHCWs should receive HIV vaccinations to avoid potential contraction of hepatitis B virus.

CLINICAL APPLICATION

With a peer evaluating your performance, prepare a treatment room for patient care. Follow OSHA and other guidelines that are specific to your treatment facility.

CRITICAL-THINKING ACTIVITIES

Evaluate the following scenarios, and make corrections as you deem necessary to meet standard operating procedure.

1. You are short of time in preparing the treatment room for the patient, and with a single spray you quickly wipe down the handpiece with a surface disinfectant. While scrubbing your hands, you notice that you have an open cut on your left hand, but it is not painful. You decide not to wear latex gloves because the patient is a family member who has been seen as a patient of record. You seat the patient and proceed to provide treatment as directed by the operator.

2. Recently, you have had a "cold," and suddenly you have the urge to sneeze. You turn away, sneeze, and blow your nose. Treatment continues and you pass the operator the next instrument. An instrument, that is not on the tray setup is needed. You quickly open the drawer of the mobile cart to retrieve the instrument. While you are doing this, the HVE tip slips out of the hose onto the floor. You know it is the last tip in the room, so you retrieve it and continue to evacuate the oral cavity.

9   Dental Radiography

LEARNING OBJECTIVES

You will have mastered the material in this chapter when you can:

- Define the key terms
- Describe how x-ray photons are produced in a radiographic machine
- List and identify equipment components that limit and control excessive exposure to ionizing radiation in dentistry
- Define the ALARA concept
- List and identify procedures used to minimize exposure to ionizing radiation
- Observe the patient's reaction and modify the procedure to ensure patient comfort throughout the radiographic examination
- Answer patient safety questions or concerns based on knowledge, facts, and scientific data
- Describe the process by which radiographic images are created
- Describe the film placement and angle of projection used in the two major intraoral techniques (bisecting and paralleling)
- Differentiate between the types of radiographic films and
  how they are used in dentistry
- Select the appropriate film and correctly position it for all periapical and bite-wing projections
- Define radiographic characteristics of density, contrast, geometric unsharpness, magnification, and shape distortion
- List the visual characteristics of an acceptable radiograph
- List and explain the quality control procedures necessary in dental radiography
- Evaluate radiographs for technical and diagnostic quality; determine whether retake or additional radiographs are required for adequate diagnostic evaluation of the region of interest
- Given a radiograph of poor quality, identify and explain the cause and correction of errors
- Describe how dental radiographic film is developed

- Explain automatic and manual processing procedures
- Explain the process of film duplication used in dentistry.
- Explain the legal factors involved in exposing, transferring and retaining dental radiographs

KEY TERMS

Anode
As low as reasonably achievable (ALARA)
Atoms
Bisecting technique
Bite-wing (BW)
Bremsstrahlung
Cathode
Cephalogram
Characteristic radiation
Collimation
Electrons
Energy
Epilation
Erythema
Exposure
Filtration
Gray
Kilovolt peak (kVp)
Kinetic Energy
Matter
Maximum permissible dose (MPD)
Milliampere (mA)
Occlusal radiograph
Panoramic
Paralleling technique
Periapical radiograph (PA)
Position-indicating device (PID)
Quality assurance
Rad
Radiation
Radiation safety
Radiograph
Radiology
Radiolucent
Radiopaque
Rem
Selective absorption

Sievert
Target
Tube head
X-ray

FILL-IN QUESTIONS

1. Why is a complete intraoral radiographic examination so important to a dental diagnosis? Explain what can be seen in this type of examination that cannot be seen in an intraoral visual examination.

2. Define a full-mouth radiographic survey.

3. What is the function of a periapical radiograph?

4. What is the function of a bite-wing radiograph?

5. List the anatomic structures visible in a:
   a. Periapical:

   b. Bite-wing:

6. Define the purpose of using a vertical rather than a horizontal bite-wing.

7. In space provided draw a mesial view of a maxillary premolar with film packet in place. Place a line between the film packet and tooth to indicate the basic parallel concept.

8. Explain the basic principle of the bisecting technique, that is, the relationship of film packet to tooth.

From the following radiographs explain the error in exposure or processing and how it can be corrected.

FIG. 9-1 through 9-8 Radiographs.

9.

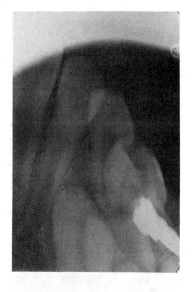

10.

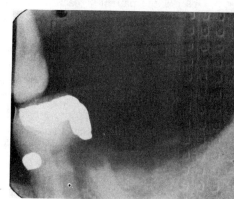

11.

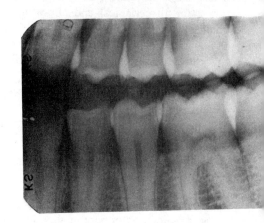

12.

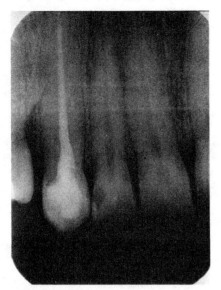

14.

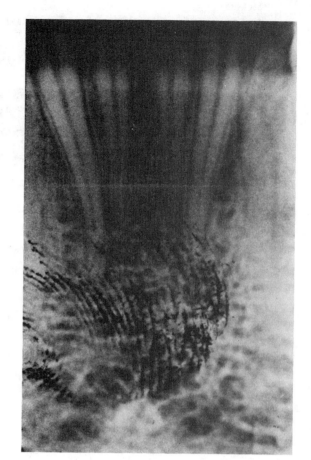

13.

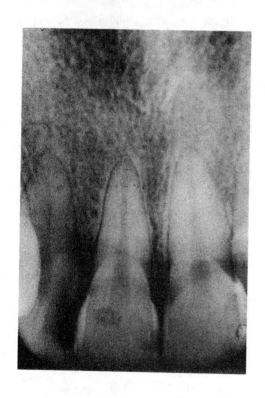

15.

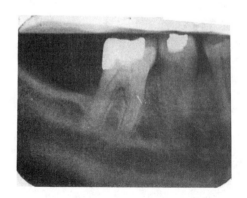

16.

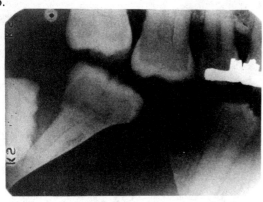

17. List the information found on a film packet:

18. List the advantages and disadvantages of panoramic radiography.

   Advantages

   Disadvantages

19. Describe the buccal object rule and why it may be necessary.

20. If a patient transfers to another dental office and asks for his or her radiographs to be forwarded to that office, you should send
   a. The original radiographs as requested.
   b. A copy of the radiographs, and keep the original as a part of the patient's permanent record.
   c. Neither the original nor a copy of radiographs, since the patient in no longer coming to your office for treatment.

21. An atom is composed of which of the following particles?
   1. Protons
   2. Neutrons
   3. Gamma rays
   4. Electrons

   a. 1, 2, and 3
   b. 1, 2, and 4
   c. 2, 3, and 4

22. Inside the radiography tube the tungsten filament is heated to produce free electrons. What is this process called?
   a. Electron generation
   b. Thermionic emission
   c. Conductivity
   d. Threshold exposure

23. To protect the patient and health care worker, which material is used in the dental x-ray tube head, film packet, and protective apron to stop x-rays?
   a. Aluminum
   b. Lead
   c. Copper
   d. Tungsten

24. When exposing a dental film to increase the number of x-rays produced, you would increase
   a. Kilovoltage
   b. Exposure time
   c. Milliamperage

25. On a radiographic film, contrast is the
   a. Magnification of the image on the film
   b. Amount of difference between the black and white area of the film
   c. Amount of penumbra on the film
   d. Degree of blackening on the film

26. An amalgam restoration appears white on a dental radiographic film. This image is referred to as
    a. Radiolucent
    b. Radiopaque
    c. Contrast

27. When a dental film is exposed, the amount of enlargement of the image on the film is controlled by the
    a. Definition
    b. Milliamperage and exposure time
    c. Source-to-film and film-to-object distance

28. A patient is seen who has recently begun treatment for cancer and is receiving oral radiation therapy. Which of the following may be side effects to the treatment?
    a. Ulcers in the mouth
    b. Cervical decay
    c. Difficulty in swallowing
    d. Leukemia
    e. Thyroid cancer

29. Small, negatively charged particles are called
    a. Atoms
    b. Electrons
    c. Protons
    d. Neutrons

30. Small, positively charged particles are called
    a. Atoms
    b. Electrons
    c. Protons
    d. Neutrons

31. A dense material that absorbs x-rays, thereby appearing light on the radiographic film, is said to be
    a. Radiolucent
    b. Radiopaque
    c. Irradiated
    d. Phosphorescent

32. A thin material that allows x-rays to pass through and thereby appears dark on the radiographic film is said to be
    a. Radiolucent
    b. Radiopaque
    c. Irradiated
    d. Phosphorescent

33. Which of the following statements is true for the focusing cup?
    1. It aims the electrons at the target.
    2. It is made of tungsten.
    3. It is made of molybdenum.
    4. It is found in the anode.
    5. It is found in the cathode.

    a. 1, 2, and 5
    b. 1, 3, and 4
    c. 1, 3, and 5
    d. 3 and 5

34. Certain organs and tissues have been designated as "critical" because they are exposed to more radiation than others. Which of the following are included in the "critical organ theory"?
    1. Mature bone
    2. Blood forming tissue
    3. Eye
    4. Thyroid
    5. Kidneys

    a. 1, 2, and 3
    b. 1, 3, and 4
    c. 2, 3, and 4
    d. 2, 3, and 5
    e. 1, 3, and 5

35. When negative angulation is used for examination of the mandibular teeth, the PID will be pointing
    a. Up
    b. Down
    c. Perpendicular

36. When positive angulation is used for examination of the maxillary teeth, the PID will be pointing
    a. Up
    b. Down
    c. Perpendicular

37. Bite-wing radiographs are taken at _____ angulation in both the bisecting and the paralleling techniques.
    a. Zero
    b. Plus 10
    c. Negative 10
    d. Plus 50

38. In the paralleling technique the film-to-tooth distance must be _____ to keep the film parallel to the tooth.
    a. Increased
    b. Decreased
    c. Altered

39. Poor horizontal angulation for a bite-wing film will result in
    a. Foreshortening
    b. Overlapping of image
    c. Elongating of image
    d. Elongating of roots

40. Cone cutting results in an unexposed area on the film. To correct this situation
    a. Decrease vertical angulation.
    b. Change position of patient's occlusal plane.
    c. Align central x-ray beam with the center of the film.

CLINICAL APPLICATIONS

1. With a radiographic manikin and unit, expose, process, and mount a full-mouth series of radiographs. Evaluate the quality of the radiographs, review them with your instructor, and identify errors. For unacceptable films, repeat film exposures until you achieve 100% competency.

2. Obtain an unmounted, full series of radiographs from your instructor. Mount the radiographs, and on a sheet of paper describe and list all anatomic features that are visible on each film.

CRITICAL THINKING ACTIVITIES

1. A patient who is in the first trimester of a pregnancy is scheduled to have a complete radiographic series. The patient informs you that she wishes not to have this treatment. How should you respond? If the treatment for this patient had been an emergency, with the patient experiencing severe discomfort and requiring a single periapical film exposure would you have responded differently? Explain your answer.

2. A 72-year-old male patient who is seen biannually in the office is asymptomatic and is scheduled to have a complete series of radiographs, 14 periapicals and 4 bite-wings. His last complete radiographs were taken 5 years ago. He states that he cannot afford this treatment now and wants to know if there is an alternative.

3. A 42-year-old female patient with extensive previous restorative treatment is displaying visual evidence of periodontal disease. Her last complete dental radiographs were taken by another dentist 4 or 5 years ago. The dentist has prescribed a complete series of radiographs. She questions you about why she should have these x-rays and wonders if you couldn't take "one of those x-rays that circle around the head." Explain your response. What action could be taken?

10 Pharmacology

LEARNING OBJECTIVES

You will have mastered the material in this chapter when you can:

- Define the key terms
- Give the definition for a drug
- Discuss current drug legislation
- Define the terms *trade name, generic name,* and *generic equivalent*
- List the sources of accurate drug information
- Define and discuss drug interaction, reactions, and effects
- List and discuss the types of drugs used in dentistry
- Describe the parts of a prescription
- Describe and discuss how to take or update a drug and allergy history
- Discuss the dental assistant's responsibilities for drugs used in dental practice
- Discuss the dental assistant's responsibilities when an emergency occurs
- Discuss important areas of patient education

KEY TERMS

Allergic
Analgesic
Anaphylactic
Angioedema
Antagonistic
Antibiotic
Antibody
Antigen
Antihistamine
Antineoplastic
Antiseptic
Barbiturate
Contraindications
Drug Enforcement Agency (DEA)
Food and Drug Administration (FDA)
Generic
Generic equivalent
Germicide
Hemostatic agent
Hypnotic

Illegal drug
Intradermal
Intramuscular (IM)
Intravenous (IV)
Legal drug
Narcotic
National Formulary (NF)
Nonprescription
Parenteral
Physicians' Desk Reference (PDR)
Pharmacology
Prescription
Sedative
Subcutaneous (SC)
Synergistic
Topical
Trade name
Tranquilizer
United States Pharmacopoeia (USP)
Vasoconstrictor

FILL-IN QUESTIONS

1. If a patient is having difficulty or distress in breathing, he or she is said to be suffering from:

   _____.

2. Tachycardia is a _____ heart beat; bradycardia is a _____ heart beat.

3. List the drug reference texts commonly used during treatment of patients

   _____

   _____

   _____

4. List the four main categories of drugs used in a dental practice.

_____

_____

_____

_____

5. If a drug is considered a generic drug, the name is:

_____.

6. If a drug is designated by a trade name, the name is:

_____.

MATCHING QUESTIONS

Match each of the following terms with the correct description.

_____ 7. Antagonistic	a.	Drug that depresses the CNS
_____ 8. Germicide		
_____ 9. PDR	b.	Within a muscle
_____ 10. FDA	c.	Within the skin
_____ 11. USP	d.	Organic compounds that depress the CNS
_____ 12. Sedative		
_____ 13. Subcutaneous		
_____ 14. Intradermal	e.	Agent that soothes
_____ 15. Intramuscular	f.	Drug derived from opium
_____ 16. Narcotic	g.	That which counteracts the action of something else
	h.	Reference text
	i.	One of a group of antibiotics
	j.	Federal regulatory agency
	k.	Pharmacopoeia reference
	l.	Beneath the skin
	m.	Destroys microorganisms

Match each of the following terms with the correct description.

_____ 17. qh	a.	Three times a day
_____ 18. stat	b.	With water
_____ 19. qod	c.	By mouth
_____ 20. cap	d.	As desired
_____ 21. ad lib	e.	Before meals
_____ 22. ac	f.	Take every hour
_____ 23. tid	g.	Every day
_____ 24. pc	h.	Twice a day
	j.	After a meal
	k.	Capsule
	l.	Every other day
	m.	Immediately
	n.	Every 2 hours

MULTIPLE-CHOICE QUESTIONS

25. Anaphylactic shock results from
   a. A reaction to mental depression
   b. Sudden, violent allergic reaction
   c. Aspiration of a foreign object
   d. A chronic allergic reaction

26. Parenteral may refer to all routes of administration *except*
   a. Subcutaneous
   b. Intramuscular
   c. Intravenous
   d. Oral

27. Factors influencing drug action that must be considered when prescribing a drug for a patient include
   1. Weight
   2. Height
   3. Gender
   4. Age

   a. 1 and 3
   b. 1, 2, and 3
   c. 1, 3, and 4
   d. 1, 2, 3, and 4

28. Modifications in dental therapy for the asthmatic patient may include
   a. Stress and anxiety reduction
   b. Requiring patient to bring his or her bronchodilator to the dental appointment
   c. Use of nitrous oxide to relieve anxiety
   d. Both a and b
   e. None of the above

29. Examples of psychosedation before and during dental treatment include
    a. Use of calming medications
    b. Use of nitrous oxide before administration of local anesthetic possibly during treatment
    c. Administration of local anesthetic for pain control
    d. Both a and b
    e. All of the above

30. A patient's medical history reveals that he has a seizure disorder, and an oral examination reveals that fibrous hyperplasia exists. Which of the following drugs might this patient be taking?
    a. Tetracycline
    b. Megadoses of iron supplement
    c. Dilantin
    d. Amoxicillin

31. A dentist wants a patient to take a prescribed drug three times a day. The prescription might contain which of the following in the signa?
    a. Take one capsule TID.
    b. Take one capsule q8h
    c. Take one capsule with breakfast, with dinner, and at bedtime.
    d. All of the above
    e. Only a

32. The following signa appears on a prescription: Amoxicillin 500 mg q12h Refill 0. The patient will
    1. Take the drug two times a day
    2. Take the drug four times a day
    3. Refill the prescription once
    4. Be able to stop taking the medication when feeling better
    5. The patient will not be able to refill the prescription.

    a. 2
    b. 1 and 5
    c. 1, 4, and 5
    d. 2 and 4
    e. 2, 4, and 5

CLINICAL APPLICATION

Why is it important for the dentist to have complete information regarding prescription and nonprescription drugs that a patient takes on a regular basis?

CRITICAL-THINKING ACTIVITY

A patient came to you while the dentist was not in the office and was concerned about a drug that had been prescribed. What source would you be able to refer to in obtaining information for this patient? What information would you be able to give the patient?

11 Dental Materials

LEARNING OBJECTIVES

You will have mastered the material in this chapter when you can:

- Define the key terms
- Explain the purpose of dental materials
- List the organizations responsible for establishing standards and specifications for dental materials
- Describe the properties of dental materials
- Identify the relationship of infection control and hazardous substances to dental materials
- Identify preventive dental materials
- Explain the function of preventive dental materials
- Describe the manipulation of preventive dental materials
- Identify direct restorative dental materials
- Explain the function of direct restorative dental materials
- Describe the manipulation of direct restorative dental materials
- Identify indirect restorative dental materials
- Explain the function of indirect and adjunct restorative dental materials
- Describe the manipulation of indirect restorative dental materials
- Identify and explain the sequence of use for finishing, polishing, and cleansing materials

KEY TERMS

Base
Compressive strength
Corrosion
Council on dental materials, instruments, and equipment
Deformation
Dimensional change
Direct
Ductile
Electrical properties
Exothermic reaction
Flow
Force
Galvanism
Hardness
Heavy body
Indirect
Light body
Luting
Malleable
Mechanical properties
Percolation
Primary consistency
Retentive properties
Secondary consistency
Shear strength
Solubility and sorption
Strain
Stress
Syneresis
Tensile strength
Thermal conductivity
Viscosity
Wettability
Yield point

FILL-IN QUESTIONS

Classify the following impression materials as rigid (R) or elastic (E).

_____ 1. Agar hydrocolloid
_____ 2. ZOE impression paste
_____ 3. Dental compound
_____ 4. Alginate hydrocolloid
_____ 5. Impression plaster
_____ 6. Polysulfide
_____ 7. Polyether
_____ 8. Addition silicone
_____ 9. Condensation silicone
_____ 10. Agar/alginate hydrocolloid

11. Which of the impression materials listed above are reversible?

_____

12. When a restorative material is being selected for use in the oral cavity, certain physical and biological factors should be considered. List four of these factors (physical or biological), and explain why they are important.

Factor

a. _____

b. _____

c. _____

d. _____

Reason for concern

a. _____

b. _____

c. _____

d. _____

13. List five uses of plastics in dentistry.

a. _____

b. _____

c. _____

d. _____

e. _____

14. In the formation of plastic the reaction involves the combination of single molecules called _____ into chains of molecules called _____. The reaction is called _____.

15. Dental amalgam alloy is mixed with _____ to form a dental restorative material.

16. List the three phases that are formed during the setting reaction of dental amalgam, and explain the components of each phase.

Phase

a. _____

b. _____

c. _____

Components of phase

a. _____

b. _____

c. _____

17. State two functions of condensation.

_____

_____

18. Gold alloys used in dentistry are referred to as "cast metal". Explain the term *cast metal*, and briefly describe how this type of restoration is used.

19. The four goals in restorative dentistry are to restore the tooth as follows:

a. _____

b. _____

c. _____

d. _____

MATCHING QUESTIONS

Match each of the following terms with the statement that best describes it.

a. Microleakage
b. Ductility
c. Adhesion
d. Strain
e. Corrosion

e. Solubility
f. Flow
g. Cohesion
h. Elasticity
i. Stress
j. Galvanism
k. Malleability
l. Ultimate strength

20. _____ Ability of a material to dissolve in solution
21. _____ Change in the length of a material as a result of force
22. _____ Point at which a material will fracture or rupture at a certain stress
23. _____ Ability of a material to withstand permanent deformation under a compressive stress
24. _____ Ability of a material to move across a surface
25. _____ Ability of a material to withstand deformation under tensile stress
26. _____ Battery effect produced by two different metals
27. _____ Process whereby the surface of a material becomes rough and pitted by going into solution
28. _____ Measure of the amount of deformation in a material under a constant load
29. _____ Movement of fluids and microorganisms into the space between the cavity preparation and the restoration
30. _____ Property of a material that permits it to be deformed under stress and then assume its original configuration when the stress is removed
31. _____ Force that causes like molecules to attach to one another
32. _____ Force that causes unlike molecules to attach to one another

MULTIPLE-CHOICE QUESTIONS

33. Which of the following statements is (are) true?
    1. An impression gives a negative reproduction of a tooth.
    2. An impression gives a positive reproduction of the soft tissue.
    3. The die of a mandibular molar is a positive duplication of the tooth.
    4. The die of a maxillary molar is a negative duplication of the tooth.
       a. 1 and 3
       b. 2 and 4

c. 1, 2, and 3
d. 4 only

34. Tearing of rubber impression materials when removing them from the mouth can be minimized by
    a. Use of an alginate material instead
    b. Allowing the impression to remain in the mouth an additional 2 minutes
    c. Removal with a rapid, uniform motion

35. Which of the following is a test for measuring hardness?
    a. Resilience
    b. Toughness
    c. Thompson
    d. Knoop

36. If a dimensional change occurs in an impression to be used to create a restoration, the following can happen; it can
    1. Result in shrinkage of the impression material.
    2. Result in the expansion of the impression material.
    3. Affect the accuracy of the dental restoration.
    4. Affect the thermal coefficient of expansion of the material.

    a. 1 and 3
    b. 2 and 4
    c. 1, 2, and 3
    d. 4 only

37. Cavity varnish is used to
    1. Seal dentinal tubules
    2. Provide an anodyne effect
    3. Seal margins of cavity preparations
    4. Provide insulation

    a. 1 and 3
    b. 2 and 4
    c. 1, 2, and 3
    d. 4 only

38. Syneresis refers to the following:
    a. Intake of fluid
    b. Loss of fluid

39. An accelerator added to a dental material will
    a. Increase the working or setting time
    b. Decrease the working or setting time

40. An increase in the water proportion of a gypsum product can
    1. Decrease the compressive strength
    2. Increase the compressive strength
    3. Decrease the setting time
    4. Increase the setting time

    a. 1 and 3
    b. 2 and 4
    c. 1 and 4
    d. 2 and 3

41. An indirect technique for constructing a cast gold alloy restoration means that the following are true:
    1. A final impression is made of the prepared tooth.
    2. A final impression is not made of the prepared tooth.
    3. The wax pattern is made on the prepared tooth.
    4. The wax pattern is made on the die.

    a. 1 and 3
    b. 2 and 3
    c. 1 and 4
    d. 1,2, and 3

42. When the frozen slab technique is used in mixing zinc phosphate cement, the following is true:
    a. Setting time is increased.
    b. Setting time is decreased.

43. Which is the correct sequence of events for creating a gold alloy casting?
    a. Making the wax pattern, creating the die, investing the pattern, spruing the pattern, burnout, casting, and pickling
    b. Creating the die, making the wax pattern, spruing the pattern, investing the wax pattern, burnout, casting, and pickling
    c. Creating the die, making the wax pattern, spruing the pattern, investing the wax pattern, casting, burnout, and pickling
    d. Creating the wax pattern, spruing the die, investing the wax pattern, pickling, casting, and burnout

44. Which of the following is not true about porcelain in dentistry?
    a. It is used as an intracoronal restoration and is inserted directly into the tooth like a composite restoration.
    b. It is more translucent than other materials.
    c. It is well tolerated by oral tissues.
    d. It is used for denture teeth, facings, laminates, and fusion to gold alloys.

45. Which of the following statements is not true regarding finishing, polishing, and cleansing materials used in dentistry?
    a. Abrasives vary in grits.
    b. The pressure exerted on an abrasive changes the rate of abrasion.
    c. Abrasives are always supplied as disposables.
    d. Polishing agents are supplied in a variety of grits.

46. The gold content of an 18-K alloy is:
    a. 80%
    b. 50%
    c. 75%
    d. 100%

47. Which of the following statements describes the purpose of the specifications of the American National Standards Institute and the American Dental Association?
    1. The specifications measure clinical properties of materials to establish minimum standards.
    2. The specifications measure critical physical and mechanical properties of materials to establish minimum standards.
    3. Lists of certified materials ensure clinical success.
    4. Lists of certified materials ensure quality control and are helpful in selection of dental materials for a dental practice.

    a. 1 and 3
    b. 2 and 4
    c. 1 only
    d. 4 only

48. Which of the following restorative materials have values of thermal conductivity similar to those of human enamel and dentin?
   1. dental amalgam
   2. composite plastics
   3. gold alloys
   4. zinc phosphate cement

   a. 1 and 3
   b. 2 and 4
   c. 1, 2, and 3
   d. 4 only

49. Which of the following are examples of galvanism in restorative dentistry?
   1. A piece of plastic wrap becomes wedged between two teeth and contacts a gold restoration.
   2. A temporary aluminum crown contacts a gold restoration.
   3. A temporary plastic crown contacts a gold restoration.
   4. A metallic taste is a frequent complaint of a patient.

   a. 1 and 3
   b. 2 and 4
   c. 1, 2, and 3
   d. 4 only

50. Which of the following conditions could lead to corrosion in restorative dentistry?
   1. A chemical attack of a metal by components in food or saliva
   2. Polished amalgams that have become dull and discolored with time
   3. Adjacent restorations constructed of dissimilar metals

   a. 1 and 3
   b. 1, 2 and 3
   c. 2 only

51. Linear coefficient of thermal expansion is a measure of the
   a. Amount of heat transferred through a material
   b. Biting force a material can withstand
   c. Change in size of a material resulting from changes in temperature
   d. pH of a material

52. Etching of the tooth surface is done primarily with
   a. Phosphoric acid
   b. Acetic acid
   c. Hydrochloric acid
   d. Nitric acid

53. Pit and fissure sealants are retained on the tooth surface by
   a. Mechanical lock
   b. Chemical bonding
   c. Adhesion
   d. Cohesion

54. Fluoride is most effective in reducing
   a. Pit and fissure caries
   b. Mottling
   c. Smooth surface caries
   d. Osteoradionecrosis

55. Which of the following would not be true for an undermixed amalgam?
   a. It has greater strength than normal.
   b. It is a dry, crumbly mass.
   c. It has lesser strength than normal.
   d. It has a dull appearance.

56. Which of the following safety measures should be followed when working with mercury?
   1. Mercury should not be handled by bare skin.
   2. Spills should be vacuumed up immediately.
   3. Mercury and amalgam scrap should be placed in the trash.
   4. Spills should be cleaned up with a special spill kit.
   5. Mercury and amalgam scrap should be stored in capped, unbreakable jars.

   a. 1, 2, and 5
   b. 2 and 3
   c. 1, 3, and 5
   d. 1, 4, and 5

57. Which of the following safety measures should also be followed when working with mercury?
   1. Reusable mixing capsules are preferred.
   2. When old amalgam restorations are being removed, water spray and high-volume evacuation should be used.
   3. When old amalgam restorations are being removed, a face mask should be worn.
   4. Single-use capsules are preferred.
   5. Operatories should be carpeted.

   a. 2, 3, and 4
   b. 2, 4, and 5
   c. 1, 3, and 4
   d. 2, 3, 4, and 5

58. Hygroscopic expansion results from
   a. Temperature increases
   b. Temperature decreases
   c. Addition of water
   d. Removal of water

59. $ZnPO_4$ contains:
   a. Reinforced ZOE
   b. Zinc polycarboxylate
   c. Phosphoric acid
   d. Calcium hydroxide

60. Zinc phosphate is mixed over a large area of the glass slab to
   a. Dissipate the heat from the reaction
   b. Thin the mix
   c. Speed up the reaction
   d. Remove excess water

61. The major disadvantage of zinc phosphate cement is that it is
   a. Too thin
   b. Too weak
   c. Too acidic
   d. Difficult to place

62. An obtundent material is one that is
   a. Drying
   b. Soothing
   c. Cleansing
   d. Irritating

63. The weakest of the gypsum products is
   a. Dental plaster
   b. Dental stone
   c. Improved dental stone

64. Which of the following waxes is considered a pattern wax?
   1. Baseplate wax
   2. Inlay wax
   3. Sticky wax
   4. Casting wax
   5. Boxing wax

   a. 1, 2, and 4
   b. 2, 4, and 5
   c. 2, 3, and 4
   d. 2 only

65. Which of the following statements are true about ZOE cements?
   1. They should be used under composite restorations.
   2. Increases in temperature and humidity will shorten setting time.
   3. They may be used under amalgam restorations.
   4. They may be used during pulp capping procedures.
   5. It is the strongest for permanent cementation.

   a. 2 and 3
   b. 2, 3, and 4
   c. 1, 2, 3, and 4
   d. All are true.

66. Zinc phosphate cement is used as follows:
   1. For permanent cementation of cast gold restoration
   2. To soothe the pulp
   3. To serve as luting for orthodontic bands
   4. As thermal insulator
   5. To stimulate formation of dentin

   a. 2 and 4
   b. 1, 3, and 4
   c. 3, 4, and 5
   d. 1, 2, 3, and 4

67. Which of the following are reasons for placing a cement base? To
    1. Strengthen the tooth
    2. Serve as a thermal insulator
    3. Serve as a thermal conductor
    4. Replace missing dentin
    5. Stimulate dentin formation

    a. 2 and 4
    b. 3 and 4
    c. 1, 2, and 4
    d. 2, 4, and 5

TRUE OR FALSE QUESTIONS

Place a **T** for True or an **F** for False next to each statement.

_____ 68. Cements are used for luting of restorations and as bases.

_____ 69. Low-strength bases provide thermal protection for the pulp.

_____ 70. *Luting* and *base* are synonymous terms.

_____ 71. Zinc phosphate cements are used in near exposures because of their obtundent quality.

_____ 72. Zinc phosphate and zinc oxide-eugenol cements must be mixed rapidly to enable the operator to place the cement into the cavity preparation quickly.

_____ 73. When a polycarboxylate cement becomes stringy or starts to "cobweb," the material is no longer usable.

_____ 74. The final setting time of stone can be decreased by adding cold water,

_____ 75. *Trituration* and *mulling* are synonymous terms.

_____ 76. Moisture interferes with the retention of a sealant.

_____ 77. Percolation can cause irritation to the pulp and recurrent decay.

_____ 78. Dental compound in cake form could be used to take an impression of an edentulous arch.

_____ 79. A bite registration impression is used to reproduce a single arch of a patient's occlusion.

_____ 80. Polymerization shrinkage of composite can be reduced by placing all of the polymer into the preparation at once.

CRITICAL THINKING ACTIVITIES

1. For the past several days you have noticed that the amalgam you have been mixing is not consistent. Sometimes it is crumbly and other times it seems almost soupy. You fail to mention this to the dentist, although you notice that she seems to have difficulty in condensing the material. She asks you whether you mixed the material for the prescribed time, and you respond affirmatively. What should be done? What is your ethical responsibility in this situation? What effect will this have on the restoration?

2. An assistant in the office suggests that you are taking too much time mixing zinc phosphate cement. Typically you divide the powder into increments and add each increment to the liquid every 10 to 15 seconds, resulting in total mixing time for a base of approximately 2 to 2½ minutes. The other assistant states that if you add a lot of powder at one time and spatulate it quickly, you can mix the material in about 20 seconds. How can you justify your method?

UNIT III

The Business of Dentistry

12   Ethical and Legal Aspects of Dentistry

LEARNING OBJECTIVES

You will have mastered the material in this chapter when you can:

- Define the key terms
- Explain the importance of ethics and law to dentistry
- Differentiate between the various types of law that affect the practice of dentistry
- Explain various types of consent
- Explain the effect of the Good Samaritan Law on health care professions
- Describe the code of ethics of professional dental organizations
- Explain the importance of a state dental practice act
- Identify the function of a state board of dentistry

KEY TERMS

Abandonment
Administrative law
Assault
Assignment
Battery
Civil law
Consent
Credential
Defendant
Defamation of character
Dental practice act
Ethics
Expert witness
Fact witness
Felony
Fraud
Implied consent
Informed consent
Invasion of privacy
Law
Lawsuit
Litigation
Malpractice
Misdemeanor

Negligence
Patient of record
Plaintiff
Respondeat superior
Standard of care
Stare decisis
Statutory law
Supervision
Tort
U.S. Constitution

FILL-IN QUESTIONS

1. The two forms of consent that exist in the delivery of dental care are _____ and _____.
2. What four questions should be asked to determine an unintentional tort of negligence in dental care?

   1. _____

   2. _____

   3. _____

   4. _____

3. Identify 10 steps that should be followed when making ethical decisions.

   _____

   _____

   _____

   _____

   _____

   _____

   _____

   _____

   _____

_____

4. Identify 10 implied duties that a dentist owes a patient.

_____

_____

_____

_____

_____

_____

_____

_____

5. List 10 acts that could lead to potential negligence.

_____

_____

_____

_____

_____

_____

_____

_____

6. Define the elements of informed consent:

1. _____

2. _____

3. _____

4. _____

MATCHING

From the list below, choose the term that best identifies each of the various situations.

   a.   abandonment
   b.   assault or battery
   c.   negligence
   d.   defamation of character
   e.   fraud
   f.   false imprisonment
   g.   invasion of privacy

7. _____ Unexcused harmful or offensive physical contact intentionally performed

8. _____ A child misbehaves in a dental chair, and a dentist uses force and restraint without the consent of the parent or legal guardian.

9. _____ Failing to use appropriate sterilization techniques

10. _____ Touching of the body of a patient in an area other than the oral cavity by the dentist

11. _____ Severance of a professional relationship with a patient who is still in need of dental care and attention without giving adequate notice to the patient

12. _____ Deception deliberately practiced in order to secure unfair or unlawful gain

13. _____ Communication of false information about a person to a third party results in injury to a person's reputation

14. _____ Altering an insurance claim form for a patient who is ineligible for coverage

15. _____ Failing to do something that a reasonably prudent person would do, or doing something that a reasonably prudent person would not do

16. _____ Transferring information to an insurance company about a patient without the patient's consent

Match the following terms with the correct definitions.

17. _____ Dental practice act
18. _____ Stare decisis
19. _____ Civil law
20. _____ Criminal law
21. _____ Misdemeanor
22. _____ Felony
23. _____ Intentional
24. _____ Standard of care
25. _____ Negligence
26. _____ Malpractice
27. _____ Litigation
28. _____ Lawsuit
29. _____ Plaintiff
30. _____ Ethics
31. _____ Doctrine of respondeat superior
32. _____ Fact witness
33. _____ Defendant
34. _____ Expert witness

a. "Let the decision stand."
b. Defines the scope of dental practice and the requirements necessary to practice
c. The equipment manufacturer
d. The person or party that institutes the suite in court
e. Relates to duties between persons or between citizens and their government
f. Wrongs committed against the public as a whole
g. Treatment that a reasonable person would perform in similar circumstances
h. A less serious crime, which is punishable by a fine or imprisonment for less than a year
i. The person committing the act intended to do so
j. The performance of an act that a reasonably careful person under similar circumstances would not do, or the converse
k. More serious crime, which is punishable by imprisonment for more than a year
l. Negligence by professionals, but can mean, in a broader sense, any wrongdoing by professionals
m. The process of a lawsuit
n. Legal action in a court
o. Person being accused of the wrongdoing
p. When placed under oath, must provide only firsthand knowledge, not hearsay
q. When testifying, must explain what happened based on the patient's record and offer an opinion as to whether the dental care, as administered, met acceptable standards
r. Differentiation between right and wrong
s. Holds an employer liable for the negligent acts of an employee

MULTIPLE-CHOICE QUESTIONS

35. Risk management programs provide all *except* the following:
    a. Competent practice
    b. Aid to the dental professional in identifying, analyzing, and dealing with risks in the dental office
    c. Information on operating safety, product safety, quality assurance, and waste disposal
    d. Teaching dental professionals how to avoid exposing themselves to liability

36. The dental assistant's best legal safeguard is the following:
    a. Competent practice
    b. Liability insurance
    c. To become credentialed
    d. To be a member of a professional organization

37. Which of the following statements is *not* true regarding the Good Samaritan Law?

    a. Most states have legislation that grants immunity for acts performed by a person who renders care in an emergency situation.
    b. It serves as an incentive for health care providers to provide medical assistance to the injured in the case of an automobile accident or other disaster, without the fear of potential litigation.
    c. This law provides protection for a negligent health care provider.
    d. This law is intended for the "Good Samaritan" who does not seek compensation but rather is solely interested in providing care to the injured in a caring, safe manner with no intent to do bodily harm.

TRUE OR FALSE QUESTIONS

For the following questions place a **T** for True and **F** for False next to each question.

_____ 38. Both legal requirements and voluntary or professional standards are implemented for the protection of society, and ultimately, the patient.

_____ 39. Membership in a professional organization is voluntary, thus the standards of these organizations are considered voluntary but are used as guidelines in peer review.

_____ 40. The state boards of dentistry are responsible for the regulation of the practice of dentistry in the individual states.

_____ 41. *Credentialing* is a generic term that refers to the ways in which professionals can maintain their competence.

_____ 42. The processes used in credentialing include accreditation, certification, and licensure.

_____ 43. Consent is the voluntary acceptance of or agreement with what is planned or done by another person.

_____ 44. To examine or treat a patient without consent constitutes an unauthorized touching and makes the person committing the act guilty of battery.

13   Human Relations in the Dental Office

LEARNING OBJECTIVES

You will have mastered the material in this chapter when you can:

- Define the key terms
- Explain human relations in dentistry
- Describe Maslow's hierarchy of needs
- Describe Carl Rogers' client-centered therapy
- Explain the concept of dentistry as a service profession
- Identify desirable characteristics in building relationships
- Describe the relationship between communication and productivity
- Identify barriers to communication
- Recognize nonverbal cues
- Describe how to improve verbal images
- Define patient rights
- Explain staff management.
- Describe professional etiquette

KEY TERMS

Client centered therapy
Communication
Hierarchy of needs
Human relations
Nonverbal cues

FILL-IN QUESTIONS

1. Identify the five levels of Maslow's hierarchy, beginning with the lowest and progressing to the highest level.

   _____

   _____

   _____

   _____

   _____

2. The ability to understand and be understood is referred to as

   _____.

3. Identify 5 skills that are key to establishing good relationships.

   _____

   _____

   _____

   _____

   _____

4. Identify 5 barriers to communication.

   _____

   _____

   _____

   _____

   _____

5. List 10 rights of a patient.

   _____

   _____

   _____

   _____

   _____

   _____

   _____

6. Identify five conditions that should occur to ensure that a staff meeting is productive.

_____

_____

_____

_____

_____

_____

MULTIPLE-CHOICE QUESTIONS

7. Which of the following words should be eliminated during verbal communication in the dental office:
   a. Investment
   b. Convention
   c. Reception room
   d. Consultation

8. To become a good listener you must
   1. Listen with your eyes.
   2. Use reflective listening.
   3. Be aware of a person's feelings.
   4. Plan your response while the person is talking.
   5. Let the speaker promptly know your personal feelings .

   a. 1 and 3
   b. 2 and 4
   c. 1, 2, and 3
   d. 4 only

9. Gestures that indicate a person's inner feelings are known as
   a. Verbal cues
   b. Nonverbal cues
   c. Reflective traits

10. The most important person in the dental office is the
    a. Assistant
    b. Dentist
    c. Hygienist
    d. Patient

11. If two people are engaged in conversation and you wish to ask one of them a nonemergency type of question, you should
    1. Avoid standing within hearing range
    2. Interrupt and ask your question
    3. Leave the area and return
    4. Make a quiet noise to get their attention

    a. 1 and 3
    b. 2 and 4
    c. 1, 2, and 3
    d. 4 only

CRITICAL-THINKING ACTIVITY

1. A patient is seen in the dental office for a complete examination, diagnosis, and consultation. The dentist outlines an extensive treatment plan with no alternative treatment and explains to the patient that the cost of treatment will be about $7000. The patient indicates that he or she has no dental coverage and will not be able to have this type of treatment. The patient leaves the office and does not return. Could the patient reaction have been anticipated? Explain your response. What could have been done to prevent this reaction?

14 Business Office Procedures

LEARNING OBJECTIVES

You will have mastered the material in this chapter when you can:

- Define the key terms
- Explain the function of the dental business office
- Describe common telecommunications procedures
- Describe the effective use of an answering machine or service
- Discuss effective reception room techniques
- Identify appointment management procedures
- Differentiate between clinical and financial records
- Identify the components of a clinical record
- Identify the components of an accounts receivable system
- Explain patient record transfer
- Describe the prevention of disease transmission from the treatment room to the business office
- Identify basic types of written communication
- Explain rules for letter writing
- Describe common recall systems
- Describe the importance of inventory control
- Explain the function of dental insurance
- Describe the components of an insurance claim form
- Explain basic insurance terminology
- Describe basic filing procedures
- Describe the use of computers and other automated equipment in a dental business office

KEY TERMS

Accounts payable
Accounts receivable
Appointment schedule list
Capitation dentistry
Claim forms
Clinical chart
Clinical record
Closed panel
Code system
Coordination of benefits
Copayment
Daily journal sheet
Deductible
Facsimile (FAX)
Fixed Fee
Fraud
Informed consent form
Inventory
Laboratory requisition
Ledger card
Ledger card tray
Office policy
Predetermination
Preferred Provider Organization (PPO)
Primary carrier
Recall
Receipt/charge slip
Registration/health questionnaire
Secondary carrier
Subscriber
Table of allowance
Telecommunications
Treatment plan
Unit
Update form
Usual, customary, and reasonable (UCR)

FILL-IN QUESTIONS

1. Name the two most common bookkeeping systems used in dentistry.

   _____

   _____

2. Identify six components of a clinical record, and explain the function of each.

   Component

   _____

   Function

   _____

Component

_____

Function

_____

Component

_____

Function

_____

Component

_____

Function

_____

Component

_____

Function

_____

Component

_____

Function

_____

3. List three functions of a patient financial record.

_____

_____

_____

4. Define the function of each of the following bookkeeping materials:

a. Daily journal sheet

_____

b. Patient ledger card

_____

c. Statement

_____

d. Ledger card tray

_____

e. Super bill

_____

5. What six factors should be considered in preparing professional written communication?

_____

_____

_____

_____

_____

_____

6. Name three common types of recall systems,

_____

_____

_____

7. List eight rules for entering data on a financial record.

_____

_____

_____

_____

_____

_____

_____

8. List six rules that will enhance the processing of claim forms.

_____

_____

_____

_____

_____

9. Identify five activities that constitute fraud in insurance management.

_____

_____

_____

_____

_____

MULTIPLE-CHOICE QUESTIONS

10. What questions do you need to ask when the following call is received: "Hello, this is Mrs. Perez. I'm having some pain in a tooth and need an appointment."
    1. "May I have the correct spelling of your first and last name?"
    2. "How long has it been bothering you?"
    3. "Is it a sharp pain? Dull ache? Continuous or periodic?
    4. "What is your social security number?"
    5. "What is your birth date?"

a. 1 and 3
b. 2 and 4
c. 1, 2, and 3
d. 1, 2, 3, and 4
e. All of the above

11. When an answering machine or a professional service is used, which of the following statements applies to professional use of such techniques?
    1. Messages left on answering machines should be as caring as possible
    2. Messages left on an answering machine should indicate specific instructions as to what the patient should do in case of emergency.
    3. If an answering service is used, follow-up of messages should be as prompt as possible.
    4. Professional dental offices should use an answering service instead of a machine to provide immediate response to a problem.
    5. Professional dental offices that rely on answering machines violate basic ethics principles.

a. 1 and 3
b. 2 and 4
c. 1, 2, and 3
d. 1, 2, 3, and 4
e. 5 only

12. Transmission of information from one site to another by an electronic means is referred to as a(n)
a. FAX
b. FED EX
c. UPS
d. XEROX

13. An appointment book entry includes the
    1. Patient's complete name
    2. Treatment to be completed
    3. Business and home phone numbers
    4. Amount of time needed
    5. Cross reference, when needed

a. 1 and 3
b. 2 and 4
c. 1, 2, 3, and 4
d. All of the above

14. Accounts receivable records include
    1. Patient charges
    2. Patient payments
    3. The total monies owed the practice
    4. The total monies the dentist owes
    5. The checkbook balance

    a. 1 and 3
    b. 2 and 4
    c. 1, 2, and 3
    d. 4 and 5
    e. 5 only

15. Accounts payable refer to the
    1. Patient charges
    2. Patient payments
    3. The checkbook balance
    4. The total monies owed the practice
    5. The total monies the dentist owes

    a. 1 and 3
    b. 2 and 4
    c. 1, 2, and 3
    d. 4 and 5
    e. 5 only

16. Which of the following statements is (are) *not*
    true regarding patient financial records?
    1. They are legal documents.
    2. Each record requires neat penmanship,
       accuracy, and thoroughness in making en-
       tries.
    3. If prepared by hand, financial records are
       always written in ball point.
    4. Are subject to review by the patient as well
       as the Internal Revenue Service.
    5. Erasures may be made to the entries, if
       done neatly.

    a. 1 and 3
    b. 2 and 4
    c. 1, 2, and 3
    d. 4 and 5
    e. 5 only

17. Which of the following is not a part of accounts
    payable?
    a. Check writing
    b. Making pegboard entries
    c. Maintaining an accurate bank balance
    d. Endorsing and depositing monies
    e. Reconciling bank statements

18. When transferring patient records from the
    office to another site, the business assistant
    must do all *except*
    a. Obtain consent from the patient or legal
       representative.
    b. Retain the original record in the office.
    c. Transfer the entire record.
    d. Copy the radiographs and retain the origi-
       nals.

19. Success of a recall system is determined by:
    1. Patient education
    2. Patient motivation
    3. Consistent follow-up
    4. Type of system used

    a. 1 and 3
    b. 2 and 4
    c. 1, 2, and 3
    d. 4 only

20. Which of the following is *not* an expendable
    supply?
    a. Anesthetic needle
    b. Anesthetic syringe
    c. Dental cement
    d. Radiographic developer

21. Which of the following is *not* a capital item?
    a. Computer
    b. Curing light
    c. Surgical forceps
    d. Radiographic processor

22. Which of the following is a nonexpendable
    item?
    a. Anesthetic needle
    b. Dental cement
    c. Computer
    d. Surgical forceps

23. To avoid contamination of business records from the clinical site to the business office the dental staff should
    1. Not place records in the treatment room or near exposure to aerosols.
    2. Use overgloves when making entries.
    3. Remove contaminated gloves and wash hands before making entries.
    4. Spray the record with an OSHA-acceptable disinfectant.
    5. Not worry, since bacteria, viruses, and spores are nonevasive to paper.

    a. 1 and 3
    b. 2 and 4
    c. 1, 2, and 3
    d. 1, 2, 3, and 4
    e. 5 only

TRUE OR FALSE QUESTIONS

For the following questions place a **T** for True and **F** for False next to each question.

_____ 24. A financial record is generally kept for each patient.

_____ 25. A code system used in bookkeeping is a form of shorthand that denotes specific treatment or payments in an abbreviated form.

_____ 26. An appointment matrix is an outline of routine events in the office such as meetings, buffer periods, and holidays.

_____ 27. An appointment book entry should always be done in ink.

_____ 28. A ledger card is kept separate from the clinical record.

_____ 29. A recall system is a preventive program that recalls patients to the office for various reasons.

MATCHING QUESTIONS

Match each of the following with its definition.

_____ 30. UCR

_____ 31. Fixed fee

a. A predetermined amount is established for services rendered

_____ 32. Table of allowances

_____ 33. Capitation

b. A chart fixes a dollar amount as the benefit for each individual's dental service

c. Based on the usual, customary, and reasonable fees of the dentist

d. A dentist is paid a fixed fee per capita per month, which entitles members of a group to a specified set of services.

Match each of the following with its definition.

_____ 34. Birthday rule

_____ 35. Nonparticipating dentist

_____ 36. Certificate of eligibility

_____ 37. Claim form

_____ 38. Copayment

_____ 39. Dependent

_____ 40. Primary carrier

a. Implemented in the coordination of benefits when the patient is a dependent

b. Statement listing services rendered, date of the services, and itemization of the fees

c. Amount of percentage of the total approved amount that the subscriber is obligated to pay

d. Person, generally a spouse or child, who receives benefits of a subscriber covered by a dental plan.

e. Identification card or document verifying that the individual is covered by a particular group.

f. A dentist who has not entered into an agreement with a service corporation or an agency and has not agreed to the rules and regulations of the board of directors of the corporation

g. A dentist who has an agreement to render care to a member and dependents under the rules and regulations promulgated by a board of directors or agency

h. Proposed treatment plan submitted for verification of eligibility and identification of covered benefits, plan allowances, limitations, and exclusions

i. Dental plan that covers the patient as the employee

j. Dental plan that covers the patient as a dependent

CRITICAL-THINKING ACTIVITY

A dentist has increased the productivity in the office so much that it is necessary to add a business assistant to the office. What types of credentials should this person possess? Explain your answer.

UNIT IV

Preclinical Skills

15 Four-Handed Dentistry

LEARNING OBJECTIVES

You will have mastered the material in this chapter when you can:

- Define the key terms
- Explain the concept of advanced functions in relation to four-handed dentistry
- Describe the benefits of four-handed dentistry
- Identify the principles of motion economy
- Identify the classification of motions
- Describe six-handed dentistry
- Describe the function and styles of preset trays
- Define and explain the application of color coding
- Explain positive phrases for implementing four-handed dentistry

KEY TERMS

Classification of motion
Color coding
Ergonomics
Four-handed dentistry
Motion economy
Preset trays
Six-handed dentistry
Supine position
Work simplification

FILL-IN QUESTIONS

1. Identify the Classification of Motion patterns used in each of the following:
   Class I _____
   Class III _____
   Class V _____

2. To say that the operating team has balanced posture means that:

   _____

   _____

3. List and define the four basic principles of four-handed dentistry.

_____

_____

_____

_____

MULTIPLE-CHOICE QUESTIONS

4. Which of the following is (are) objectives(s) of four-handed dentistry?
   a. To increase productivity of the dental practice
   b. To minimize stress and fatigue
   c. To achieve high-quality dental service
   d. All of the above

5. Which of the following are required to successfully practice four-handed dentistry?
   1. Operating in a seated position
   2. Employing skilled dental auxiliaries
   3. Organization of the practice
   4. Increasing the complexity of the procedure

   a. 1 and 3
   b. 2 and 4
   c. 1, 2, and 3
   d. 1, 2, 3, and 4
   e. 4 only

TRUE OR FALSE QUESTIONS

Place a T for True or an F for False in the space provided as it relates to the statement.

_____ 6. A goal of four-handed dentistry should be to reduce the number of instruments to only those needed for the procedure at hand.

_____ 7. Preset trays are seldom used in four-handed dentistry because of the cost of instruments.

_____ 8. Class IV and V movements should be minimized in practicing four-handed dentistry

_____ 9. Work simplification results often in rearranging, eliminating, or combining and simplifying a procedure.

_____ 10. A dental auxiliary is used to transfer instruments, provide oral evacuation, prepare dental materials, and diagnose in four-handed dentistry.

_____ 11. Disorganization of treatment areas, poor appointment scheduling, and lack of standardized procedure are examples of poor time management resulting in inefficiency.

_____ 12. Efficient instrument transfer reduces a great deal of movement by the dentist.

_____ 13. Unnecessary instrument exchanges can be eliminated by using an instrument to its maximum before returning it to the assistant.

CLINICAL APPLICATION

Draw a schematically correct diagram of a treatment room designed for a right-handed operator and one for a left-handed operator. Include in the drawing all basic equipment needed to practice four-handed dentistry.

CRITICAL-THINKING ACTIVITY

Provide recommendations based on the following scenario for creating a work environment that is conducive to the principles of four-handed dentistry.

A dental office you are visiting has three treatment rooms. Two are for operative procedures, and the third is designated as the hygiene treatment room. Treatment room No. 1 is equipped with a transthorax unit, while room No. 2 has a chair with attachments on the back for head and body adjustments as well as a cuspidor.

Treatment room No. 2 has one sink and an assistant's stool with straight legs that are not mobile. The sterilization unit is kept in treatment room No. 1 so that the instruments are nearby when they are needed for a procedure. At least once a day the instruments in room No. 2 are needed in room No. 1 and the assistant retrieves the needed items.

16 The Dental Suite

LEARNING OBJECTIVES

You will have mastered the material in this chapter when you can:

- Define the key terms
- Identify the factors that determine dental office design
- Describe the basic floor plan of a dental suite
- Explain the function of each room in the dental suite
- Describe the arrangement of a dental treatment room
- Describe the basic features of dental equipment used in four-handed dentistry
- Describe office care and maintenance procedures
- Explain the use of an office evaluation form

KEY TERMS

Air/water syringe
Bracket table
Business office
Curing light
Cuspidor
Dental stool
Dental unit
Electrosurgery unit
Eyewash
Fixed cabinetry
Foot control
Handpiece
High-velocity evacuation (HVE)
Laboratory
Mobile cabinetry
Patient chair
Preset trays
Radiography processing area
Reception room
Recovery room
Treatment room
Ultrasonic scaler

FILL-IN QUESTIONS

1. List the criteria for the selection of the following:

   Operator's stool: _____

   Assistant's stool: _____

   Dental chair: _____

   Dental unit: _____

   HVE system: _____

   Fixed cabinetry: _____

   Operating light: _____

   Mobile cabinetry: _____

2. Designate the area in which each of the following might be found in a dental office.

   Omniclave: _____

   Vacuum pump: _____

   Amalgamator: _____

   Mobile cabinetry: _____

   Ultrasonic scaler: _____

   Operating light: _____

   Oral hygiene devices: _____

   Bracket table: _____

   Ultrasonic cleaner: _____

MATCHING QUESTIONS

Match the following terms with the correct definition.

_____ 3. Dentist's stool

_____ 4. Mobile cart

_____ 5. Preset tray

_____ 6. Saliva ejector

_____ 7. Dental unit

_____ 8. Operating light

_____ 9. Ultrasonic scaler

_____ 10. Supine

_____ 11. Foot control

_____ 12. Cuspidor

_____ 13. HVE

a. Device used to remove calculus mechanically
b. Must be immersed in fluid to use effectively
c. Disposal area for fluids
d. Chairside means of killing microbes
e. provides diagnosic tools
f. Raises and lowers chair
g. Movable top
h. Nose and toes parallel to floor
i. Illumination
j. Power for handpieces
k. Removes fluid from the mouth
l. Instruments for a procedure
m. Five castors
n. Handpieces housed

Match each of the following with the correct definition or activity that takes place in each location:

_____ 14. Recovery room
_____ 15. Reception room
_____ 16. Private office
_____ 17. Treatment room
_____ 18. Sterilization area
_____ 19. Business office
_____ 20. Dark room

a. Process radiographs
b. Insurance claims
c. Regain normal vital signs
d. Process instruments
e. Confidential calls
f. Children's corner
g. Dental care
h. Brush teeth
i. Mount radiographs

MULTIPLE-CHOICE QUESTIONS

21. Fiberoptic capabilities are available with
    a. Intercom systems
    b. Operating light
    c. Handpieces
    d. HVE systems

22. The following device is used to remove soft tissue during a procedure:
    a. Handpiece
    b. Electroscissor unit
    c. Fiberoptic unit
    d. Electrosurgery unit

CRITICAL-THINKING ACTIVITY

You visit a dental office for a job interview. Once in the reception room, you notice that the colors of the furniture and draperies are outdated and faded. The paint on the woodwork is chipping, there is a stale odor and when you enter the clinical area, you see evidence of bloodied cotton rolls and sponges on the floor near the wastebasket. There is a pile of syringes near the sterilizer with carpules and what appear to be contaminated needles lying nearby. What is your initial reaction? What impact does this environment have on patients?

17 Seating the Patient and Operating Team

LEARNING OBJECTIVES

You will have mastered the material in this chapter when you can:

- Define the key terms
- Explain the concept of "see ability" in dentistry
- Identify the zones of activity at chairside
- Describe the preparation of a treatment room before seating a patient
- Explain and demonstrate the process for seating a dental patient for treatment in any area of the oral cavity
- Explain and demonstrate the positioning of the assistant and operator for treatment in any area of the oral cavity
- Describe the procedure for dismissing a patient
- Explain and describe the aseptic techniques used during the setup, treatment, and dismissal of the patient
- Identify special needs of patients during the seating and dismissal procedures

KEY TERMS

Assistant's zone
Direct vision
Indirect vision
Operator's zone
Seeability
Static zone
Supine
Transfer zone
Zones of activity

FILL-IN QUESTIONS

1. Explain the zones of activity, and identify what occurs in each zone.

_____

_____

_____

_____

2. Define direct and indirect vision and give examples of when each would be used.

_____

_____

_____

_____

3. List a step-by-step procedure for seating the patient, including preparation of the room before patient entry.

_____

_____

_____

_____

_____

_____

4. List five rules that the operating team should follow to assure proper positioning:

_____

_____

_____

_____

_____

MULTIPLE-CHOICE QUESTIONS

5. The static zone is reserved for
   a. The assistant
   b. Transfer of instruments
   c. The patient
   d. None of the above

6. To reduce fatigue and stress, the operating team should sit
   a. With back straight
   b. With minimal bending at the neck
   c. With shoulders and thighs parallel to the floor
   d. All of the above

TRUE OR FALSE QUESTIONS

Place a **T** for True or an **F** for False in the space provided as it refers to statement.

_____ 7. In a supine position a patient's legs and head should be at the same level.

_____ 8. The operator's zone for a right-handed dentist is from 8 to 12 o'clock.

_____ 9. The static zone for a left-handed operator is from 12 to 2 o'clock.

_____ 10. The assistant's zone changes depending on which arch is being treated.

_____ 11. A distance of 4 to 6 inches between the operator's nose and the patient's oral cavity should be maintained to avoid encroaching on the patient's breathing space.

_____ 12. Once the patient is in a supine position and the operating team is seated, the chair base is lowered to place the head of the patient into the lap of the dentist.

_____ 13. The assistant's stool is placed as close to the patient chair as possible.

_____ 14. The assistant's legs are at a right angle to the patient's chair when the assistant is properly seated.

_____ 15. When seated, the assistant should be 4 to 6 inches higher than the operator.

CLINICAL APPLICATION

You have just directed the patient into the treatment room and are ready to seat him. Explain what you would have done before the patient's entrance, and continue to describe how you would seat this patient for treatment on tooth 30MO.

CRITICAL-THINKING ACTIVITY

An older adult patient is being seen for the first time in the office. He says he has never had dentistry performed on him while he was lying down and does not intend to start today. What would your explanation be to this patient, and how might you accommodate his needs?

18 Basic Dental Instruments

LEARNING OBJECTIVES

You will have mastered the material in this chapter when you can:

- Define the key terms
- Identify the parts of a dental instrument
- Explain the G. V. Black instrument nomenclature
- Classify dental instruments according to use
- Identify and explain the function of basic dental instruments
- Identify and describe basic hand cutting instruments
- Identify and describe supplementary instruments and armamentarium common to most dental procedures
- Explain the process of instrument sharpening

KEY WORDS

Binangle
Blade
Cone socket handle
Cutting edge
Double ended (DE)
Handle
Instrument formula
Instrument number
Monangle
Shaft
Shank
Single ended (SE)
Triple angle

FILL-IN QUESTIONS

1. Name four shanks in which handcutting instruments may be supplied.

   _____

   _____

   _____

   _____

2. State three purposes for the use of a dental mouth mirror.

   _____

   _____

   _____

MATCHING QUESTIONS

Match each of the following instruments with a function that it performs.

_____ 3. Spoon excavator
_____ 4. Hatchet
_____ 5. Hoe
_____ 6. 5C carver
_____ 7. Ward's carver
_____ 8. Small condensor
_____ 9. Explorer
_____ 10. Perio probe
_____ 11. Curet scaler
_____ 12. Ball burnisher
_____ 13. Thumb forcep
_____ 14. Plastic instrument

a. Used in a push action to remove unsupported enamel
b. Used to retrieve devices from the mobile cart
c. Used for smooth-carved amalgam anatomy
d. Used in a pushing action to remove tooth structure
e. Used to remove carious debris
f. Used to condense last increment of amalgam
g. Used to check pocket depth
h. Used to place cement
I. Used to remove calculus
j. Used to check for caries
k. Used for anatomical burnishing
l. Used to compress first increment of amalgam
m. Used to carve smooth surfaces
n. Used to carve final anatomy

MULTIPLE-CHOICE QUESTIONS

15. Which of the following instruments has (have) a four-numbered instrument formula?
    1. Angle former
    2. Enamel hatchet
    3. Gingival marginal trimmer
    4. Chisel

    a. 1 and 3
    b. 2 and 4
    c. 3 only
    d. 4 only

16. Which instrument has a standard and reversed bevel?
    a. Enamel hatchet
    b. Wedelstaedt chisel
    c. Spoon excavator
    d. Gingival marginal trimmer

17. A gingival marginal trimmer is used to place bevels as follows:
    1. On the proximal cervical floor
    2. On the axial wall
    3. On the point angle
    4. On the pulpal floor

    a. 1 and 3
    b. 1 and 4
    c. 1 only
    d. 4 only

18. Which instrument is used to remove soft debris from a cavity preparation?
    a. Angle former
    b. Gingival marginal trimmer
    c. Spoon excavator
    d. Wedelstaedt chisel

19. Which of the following instruments is considered a basic setup for most dental procedures?
    1. Cotton pliers
    2. Oral evacuator
    3. Explorer
    4. Dental floss
    5. Mouth mirror
    6. Thumb forceps

    a. 1, 3, and 5
    b. 1, 3, 5, and 6
    c. 2 and 3
    d. 2, 3, and 4

TRUE OR FALSE QUESTIONS

Place a **T** for True or an **F** for False in the space provided as it refers to each of the statements.

_____ 20. The larger the manufacturer's number on a handcutting instrument, the larger the instrument formula.

_____ 21. A DE spoon would supply both right and left working ends

_____ 22. A DE gingival marginal trimmer would supply both mesial and distal working ends.

_____ 23. A thumb forcep is used to transfer materials to and from the oral cavity.

CLINICAL APPLICATION

1. Obtain an assortment of dental instruments, and divide them into the various categories of instruments.

2. An instrument has the following notations on its handle:

   Miltex <u>10</u> - <u>80</u> - <u>7</u> - <u>12</u>   T1.
   What do each of these mean?

   Miltex _____

   10 _____

   80 _____

   7 _____

   12 _____

   T1 _____

CRITICAL-THINKING ACTIVITY

Two new assistants are hired in an office. One is a recent high school graduate with no dental experience; the other has completed an accredited dental assistant program. After a minimum amount of observation time each assistant is assigned a clinical procedure. The instruments are preset on a tray, and the procedure begins. What is the expected performance of each of these assistants if the treatment should be altered midway through the procedure? What advantages or disadvantages does each assistant face?

19   Rotary Instruments

LEARNING OBJECTIVES

You will have mastered the material in this chapter when you can:

- Define the key terms
- Describe the function of rotary devices used in dentistry today
- Explain the use of a water coolant system in conjunction with dental handpieces
- Differentiate between various types of handpieces
- Identify the various shapes, sizes, types, and functions of common rotary devices
- Describe the maintenance of handpieces

KEY TERMS

Bur
Chuck
Contraangle
Disk
Fiberoptic
Finish
Flutes
Handpiece
High speed
Low speed
Mandrel
Revolutions per minute (rpm)
Rotary
Shank
Stone

FILL-IN QUESTIONS

1. Give the common series numbers for each of the following cutting burs:

   a. Inverted cone

   _____

   b. Round

   _____

   c. Straight fissure, plain cut

   _____

   d. Straight fissure, cross cut

   _____

   e. Tapered fissure, plain cut

   _____

   f. Tapered fissure, cross cut

   _____

2. List the common types of burs that would be used for the listed functions:

   a. Remove caries

   _____

   b. Place retentive grooves

   _____

   c. Open a cavity preparation

   _____

   d. Outline a cavity preparation

   _____

   e. Place depth grooves

   _____

3. Identify the following burs:

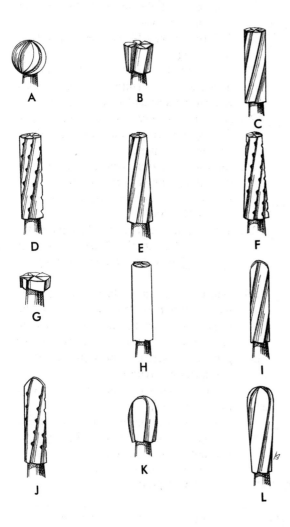

FIG. 19-1 Selection of burs.

4. If a disk is considered face in, the cutting surface is placed in what relation to the mandrel?

_____

_____

5. If a disk is considered face out, the cutting surface is in what relation to the mandrel?

_____

_____

MATCHING QUESTIONS

From the following list, select the appropriate device for each of the procedures listed below. Place the appropriate letter in the space provided. Use only one letter for each space.

a. Straight handpiece
b. Acrylic bur
c. Craytex wheel
d. Burlew disk
e. Joe Dandy disk
f. Pediatric handpiece
g. Diamond disk
h. Moore's disk
i. Prophylaxis brush
j. Screw-type mandrel
k. Bur tool
l. Moore's mandrel
m. Foot control
n. Polishing bur

_____ 6. Accepts pinhole-type disks
_____ 7. Has numerous flutes, close together
_____ 8. Attached to an angle for polishing occlusal surfaces of the teeth with a pumice-like paste
_____ 9. Is a rubberlike device used to polish gold
_____ 10. Capable of holding burs and attachments like contra angles
_____ 11. Used in the laboratory to make gross cutting as in a denture adjustment
_____ 12. Makes a "slice" on a tooth with maximum efficiency
_____ 13. Activates the handpiece
_____ 14. Tan-colored polishing device that is impregnated with pumice
_____ 15. May aid in elimination of mechanical pulp exposures
_____ 16. Made of carborundum

MULTIPLE-CHOICE QUESTIONS

17. Which of the following can be attached to a low-speed handpiece?
    1. High-speed attachment
    2. Latch-type contra angle
    3. Friction-grip bur
    4. Prophylaxis angle
    5. Latch-type bur

    a. 1 and 3
    b. 1, 2, 3, and 5
    c. 2, 3, 4, and 5
    d. All of the above

18. Which of the following can be attached to a high-speed handpiece?
    1. High-speed attachment
    2. Latch-type contra angle
    3. Friction-grip bur
    4. Prophylaxis angle
    5. Latch-type bur

    a. 1 and 3
    b. 1, 2, 3, and 5
    c. 3 only
    d. All of the above

19. Which of the following is impregnated on a bur or wheel to assist in refined tooth reduction?
    a. Carbide silicon
    b. Tungsten carbide
    c. Diamond chips
    d. Stainless steel chips

20. To open a cavity preparation, the operator would probably use the
    a. Low-speed handpiece with a straight fissure, plain cut bur
    b. High-speed handpiece with a straight fissure, plain cut bur
    c. High-speed handpiece with an inverted-cone bur
    d. Low-speed handpiece with an inverted-cone bur

TRUE OR FALSE QUESTIONS

Place a **T** for True or an **F** for false in the space provided as it refers to each of the following statements about rotary instruments.

_____ 21. The symbol **L** next to a bur number indicates that the shank is longer than the standard shank.

_____ 22. An HP bur may be used in a latch-type contra angle

_____ 23. The symbol **S** next to a bur number indicates that the cutting surface is shorter than the standard cutting surface.

_____ 24. A Moore's mandrel is a snap-on type of device that accepts only Moore's disks with metal centers.

_____ 25. Burs with a series number ¼ to 10 may be cutting burs or polishing burs.

_____ 26. A screw-type mandrel may have an RA, FG, or HP shank.

_____ 27. Water spray devices on a handpiece are used to reduce frictional heat and help to remove debris from the cavity preparation.

_____ 28. When a high-speed handpiece is used with a water coolant, it becomes the responsibility of the dental assistant to remove the accumulation of water in the patient's mouth and the water drops on the operator's mirror

_____ 29. A carborundum disk is the same device as a lightning disk.

_____ 30. Fiberoptic capabilities on a handpiece provide not only additional illumination but also increased speed.

CLINICAL APPLICATION

Take a packet of various burs, attachments, and handpieces into a treatment room, and place each on the appropraite device. Identify each item, and describe its purpose to a classmate.

CRITICAL-THINKING ACTIVITIES

1. The dentist informs you of the procedure to be completed for a patient—an amalgam core and crown preparation. Identify the burs that may be used for these procedures, and explain the purpose of each bur.

2. Compare the capabilities of current rotary devices with those of devices used 40 years ago, when only belt-driven handpieces were available in dentistry. List these capabilities, and describe the impact of this new technology on modern dentistry. Does this technology affect patients as well as the dental staff? Explain your answer.

20 Instrumentation and Exchange

LEARNING OBJECTIVES

You will have mastered the material in this chapter when you can:

- Define the key terms
- Explain the importance of instrument exchange in four-handed dentistry procedures
- Describe various instrument grasps
- Identify the basic types of instrument exchanges used at chairside
- Explain the step-by-step procedure for common instrument exchange procedures
- Describe and demonstrate how to maintain a fulcrum rest
- Describe and demonstrate the use of basic hand and rotary instruments
- Identify the responsibility of the dentist and the dental assistant during instrument exchange
- Explain various safety precautions that should be implemented during instrument exchange

KEY TERMS

Fulcrum
Hidden transfer
Instrumentation
Instrument exchange
Modified pen grasp
Palm grasp
Palm-thumb grasp
Pen grasp
Reverse exchange
Signal
Two-handed exchange

FILL-IN QUESTIONS

1. Identify three common instrument grasps.

   _____

   _____

   _____

2. When a single-handed instrument transfer technique is used, the assistant's hand is divided into two portions. Name the parts of the hand and which fingers are in each part.

   _____

   _____

3. When assisting with a right-handed dentist, the assistant passes instruments with the _____ hand and will hold the HVE in the _____ hand. Assisting a left-handed dentist requires the assistant to pass instruments with the _____ hand and use the HVE with the _____ hand.

4. Using the following outline, list the procedure for instrument passing step by step.

   I. Instrument preparation

      a. _____

      b. _____

      c. _____

      d. _____

   II. Picking up the instrument

      a. _____

      b. _____

   III. Exchanging the instrument

      a. _____

      b. _____

      c. _____

      d. _____

IV. Exceptions

    a. Mirror _____

    b. Palm grasp instruments _____

MATCHING QUESTIONS

5. Place letters of the following steps in the space provided below, to indicate the sequence of steps used in exchanging an instrument. Begin by placing the letter of the first task in the space provided for the answer to this question.

_____

    a. Place the tray as close to the patient as possible.

    b. Pick up the instrument to be transferred is with the third of the instrument nearest you.

    c. When the dentist signals, parallel the new instrument with the used instrument.

    d. Place the instruments in sequence of use on the tray.

    e. Hold the instrument to be exchanged between the thumb and first two fingers.

    f. Turn the working end of the instrument so that it is in position for the mandible or maxilla, according to the arch on which the dentist or operator is working.

    g. Grasp the used instrument with the third finger and small finger.

    h. Deliver the new instrument into the dentist's hand.

    i. If the instrument is not to be used, return the instrument to its original position on the tray.

    j. Tuck the used instrument into the palm.

    k. Roll the used instrument back into the delivery position.

For each of the following instruments select the most likely form of instrument transfer used during a dental procedure.

    a. Single-handed
    b. Two-handed
    c. Hidden syringe

_____ 6. Anesthetic syringe
_____ 7. Explorer
_____ 8. Surgical forcep
_____ 9. Scissors

_____ 10. Wedelstaedt chisel
_____ 11. Gingival marginal trimmer
_____ 12. Mirror
_____ 13. Cotton pliers
_____ 14. Surgical elevator

MULTIPLE-CHOICE QUESTIONS

15. For a right-handed operator an instrument exchange should occur
    a. In the area over the patient's mouth
    b. In the area over the patient's abdomen
    c. Where it is the easiest to gain access
    d. In the area over the patient's right shoulder
    e. In the area slightly below the patient's chin

16. When a left-handed operator is working, the preset tray should be located on the mobile cabinet in the
    a. Upper left corner
    b. Upper right corner
    c. Lower left corner
    d. Lower right corner

TRUE OR FALSE QUESTIONS

Place a **T** for True or an **F** for False in the space provided as it refers to each statement.

_____ 17. A well-organized preset tray will aid in efficient instrument transfer.

_____ 18. Pick-up of used cotton pliers is made with the pick-up fingers at the nonworking end of the pliers.

_____ 19. Effective instrument passing allows the operator to keep his or her eyes on the operative site and reduces eye strain.

_____ 20. When passing scissors, it is not necessary to parallel them with the used instrument, since there is no chance of tangling.

_____ 21. When the operator uses the a/w syringe, it is passed with the assistant holding the syringe beneath the control buttons near the hose.

_____ 22. It is necessary for the operator to adjust his or her hand position when receiving some instruments such as rubber dam forceps or scissors.

_____ 23. When it is determined that an instrument will not be needed again by the operator, it is returned to the far right side of the tray to prevent it from being used again.

_____ 24. When a maxillary right second premolar is being worked on, the working end of the instrument is placed in a downward position.
_____ 25. Instruments should never be passed over the patient's face.
_____ 26. Simultaneous delivery of the mirror and cotton pliers should occur at the beginning of most procedures.

CLINICAL APPLICATION

Practice various instrument exchanges with a classmate and a variety of instruments following the suggestions in the textbook.

CRITICAL-THINKING ACTIVITY

Imagine being confronted with the following situations during a dental procedure. Describe what might have been done to avoid the problems.

1. A bur placed in the high-speed handpiece falls out of the bur opening when the operator attempts to use it.

2. The bur is placed in the head of a high-speed handpiece, but the chuck will not completely tighten, causing slippage of the bur.

21 Oral Evacuation Systems and Techniques

LEARNING OBJECTIVES

You will have mastered the material in this chapter when you can:

- Define the key terms
- Explain the function of a high velocity evacuation system
- Explain how the HVE system can aid in reducing aerosols in a dental clinical environment
- Differentiate between the use of an HVE system and a saliva ejector
- Identify armamentarium used with an HVE system
- Explain the basic rules for oral evacuator tip placement
- Describe the placement of an evacuator tip for any given operative or surgical site
- Describe the procedure used in a complete mouth rinse
- Describe the use of the a/w syringe in maintaining a clear operating field
- Describe the routine care of the HVE system

KEY TERMS

High velocity evacuation (HVE)
Low volume evacuation (LVE)
Oral evacuation
Saliva ejector
Suction
Svedopter

FILL-IN QUESTIONS

1. State the basic rules for placement of an oral evacuator.

_____

_____

_____

_____

_____

2. Explain the method of performing a two-handed, complete mouth rinse for a patient after an operative procedure.

_____

_____

_____

_____

3. How does the procedure for a two-handed, complete mouth rinse vary from a four-handed procedure?

_____

_____

_____

4. Explain why oral evacuation is an important concept in four-handed dentistry.

_____

_____

_____

5. Explain the differences between the use of an HVE system and the use of a saliva ejector.

HVE

Saliva ejector

With a peer and a variety of instruments, practice positioning the HVE in various sites and a full-mouth rinse. Follow the suggestions in the textbook.

CRITICAL-THINKING ACTIVITIES

1. Explain the impact of the use of high-velocity evacuation on infection control.

2. A right-handed operator prepares tooth #15[3] for a restoration. Access for the handpieces is extremely limited. What possible actions could you take to accomplish the following?
   a. Remove all fluid and debris from the oral cavity.
   b. Retract the cheek from the preparation area.
   c. Maintain patient comfort.

MATCHING QUESTIONS

Choose from the list below the term that denotes the proper surface on which the suction tip is placed when the operator is using the handpiece in each of the following locations.

_____ 6. Occlusal surface   a. Labial
of #2   b. Occlusal

_____ 7. Occlusal surface   c. Lingual
of #12   d. Buccal

_____ 8. Labial surface
of #24

_____ 9. Surface 4 of #10

_____ 10. Buccal surface
of #31

_____ 11. #14[3]

_____ 12. Lingual surface
of #8

_____ 13. #19[5]

_____ 14. Lingual surface
of #19

_____ 15. Occlusal surface of #21

MULTIPLE-CHOICE QUESTIONS

16. When assisting a right-handed operator in a procedure performed on the patient's left side, the dental assistant holds the HVE tip as follows:
    a. In the right hand with a thumb-to-nose grip
    b. In the left hand with a thumb-to-nose grip
    c. In the right hand with a pen grasp
    d. In the left hand with a pen grasp

17. When assisting a left-handed operator in a procedure performed on the patient's left side, the dental assistant holds the HVE tip as follows:
    a. In the right hand with a thumb-to-nose grip
    b. In the left hand with a thumb-to-nose grip
    c. In the right hand with a pen grasp
    d. In the left hand with a pen grasp

22   Isolation Materials and Applications

LEARNING OBJECTIVES

You will have mastered the material in this chapter when you can:

- Define the key terms
- Explain the purpose of isolation techniques in dentistry
- . Identify the armamentarium used in different isolation procedures
- . Describe the step-by-step procedure in the rubber dam procedure
- . Explain the importance of rubber dam isolation in today's dentistry
- . Describe techniques in rubber dam isolation to accommodate the less ordinary oral situation

KEY TERMS

Cellulose wafer
Clamp
Clamp forceps
clamp roll holder
Frame
Hygoformics
Isolation
Ligature
Napkin
Rubber dam
Rubber dam stamp
Svedopters
Template
Winged/wingless clamps
Gingival retracting clamp
Septum

FILL-IN QUESTIONS

1. Name three basic objectives of isolation techniques.

   a. _____

   b. _____

   c. _____

2. There are a variety of devices used in dentistry for isolation. Name the two most common methods of isolation.

   a. _____

   b. _____

3. Name five types of auxiliary equipment used to retract and/or evacuate materials from the oral cavity during isolation procedures.

   a. _____

   b. _____

   c. _____

   d. _____

   e. _____

4. Using the following diagram of a rubber dam clamp, answer the following questions.

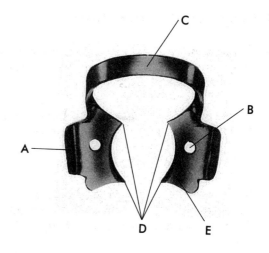

FIG. 22-1 Rubber dam clamp.

a. For what is the "A" portion of this device used?

b. For what is the "B" portion of this device used?

c. What is the general rule for placement of the "C" portion of this clamp when in proper position?

d. For what is the "D" position of this device used?

e. For what is the "E" position of this device used.

MULTIPLE-CHOICE QUESTIONS

Identify the type of clamp to be used in each of the following situations. Choose the one best answer.

_____ 5. Endodontic treatment on #8
_____ 6. Operative treatment on #9
_____ 7. Operative treatment on #29
_____ 8. Operative treatment on #5
_____ 9. Operative treatment on #14

a. Molar
b. Premolar
c. Anterior

10. Rubber dam isolation provides the following:
    1. A means of patient management
    2. Reduces stress for the operator
    3. Fluid control
    4. Control over oral tissues
    5. Reduction of microbial aerosols

    a. 1 and 4
    b. 2 and 3
    c. 3 and 5
    d. 2 only
    e. 1, 2, 3, 4, and 5

11. If a patient has a three-unit bridge in the mandibular right quadrant, the following is (are) true:
    1. The rubber dam is placed normally.
    2. The rubber dam is sewn under the pontic to reduce saliva control problems.
    3. Rubber dam isolation cannot be used.
    4. The rubber dam must be cut and pulled under the pontic.
    5. Cotton roll isolation would be the ideal isolation.

    a. 1 and 4
    b. 2 and 4
    c. 1 only
    d. 4 only
    e. 5 only

12. If treatment is to be performed on tooth #19, the following teeth would be isolated with a rubber dam:
    a. #19 through #27
    b. #18 through #27
    c. #19 through #26
    d. #18 through #30

MATCHING QUESTIONS

Select from the following elements of armamentarium the isolation material or device that meets each of the descriptions listed below.
a. Woodbury frame
b. Rubber dam clamp
c. Saliva ejector
d. Young's frame
e. Dental floss
f. Rubber dam clamp forceps
g. Spoon excavator
h. Explorer
i. Dental compound
j. Stick wax

k. Rubber dam punch
l. Svedopter
m. Celluloid wafer
n. Cotton roll holder

_____ 13. Thermoplastic material used to stabilize a Ferrier #212 or another anterior clamp
_____ 14. Device made of metal or plastic, with projections on which the rubber dam is retained
_____ 15. Plierlike instrument with a rotating table that generally includes six different sized holes
_____ 16. A material that could be used as a ligature to secure the rubber dam on the most anterior tooth
_____ 17. Metal device that is available with three tongue-retraction plates and is capable of removing fluids from the oral cavity
_____ 18. Metal instrument used in cuffing the rubber dam
_____ 19. Device that fits under the patient's chin; one side is placed around the buccal and other on the lingual of a quadrant of the mandibular arch
_____ 20. Triangular absorbent device placed in the vestibule to absorb fluid
_____ 21. Plastic or metal pronged device placed during isolation to anchor the rubber dam

CLINICAL APPLICATION

List the armamentarium necessary for the following situations.

a. Rubber dam application for operative treatment on #13MO:

b. Isolation of the mandibular right quadrant using cotton rolls.

Describe the step-by-step procedure for preparation and placement of rubber dam for isolation of #30DO.

CRITICAL-THINKING ACTIVITY

1. You are assisting in a root canal procedure on #8 tooth. How many holes do you punch in the rubber dam?

2. Operative treatment is to be provided on tooth #14$^{1-5}$. What size holes are punched? What teeth are exposed through the rubber dam?

3. You fail to place a piece of dental floss on the bow of the clamp before attaching it to the rubber dam. The operator expresses concern that the floss is not placed. Why is it important to use this floss?

4. A patient is seen for treatment on tooth #18^{MOD}. The first mandibular left molar is missing, but the third is present. On what tooth is the clamp positioned? Do you punch a hole for the missing tooth? What holes are punched?

5. A patient is about to receive treatment on tooth #2, and this tooth is the distal abutment of a bridge. Explain how you would punch the rubber dam and how you would apply it. How many holes are punched? How is it secured to avoid leakage?

6. What is the solution to each of these problems?

   a. Clamp slipping off the anchor tooth:

   b. Difficulty pulling dam through contact:

   c. Wrinkling of the dam:

   d. Rotary instruments catching dam at inter-proximal:

   e. Spaces between dam and teeth:

   f. Saliva accumulating in patient's mouth:

23 Topical and Local Anesthesia

LEARNING OBJECTIVES

You will have mastered the material in this chapter when you can:

- Define the key terms.
- Describe the purpose of anesthesia.
- Explain the different types of topical and local anesthesia and indications for use
- Describe the types of anesthesia and application in dentistry
- Explain the components of local anesthesia and the effect of each on the human body
- Identify the parts of a local anesthetic carpale/cartridge, needle, and syringe
- Describe the procedure for assembly and disassembly of the anesthetic syringe
- Identify types of syringes used in dentistry
- Explain the technique for syringe transfer
- Explain the accepted safety guidelines regarding the use of sharps

KEY TERMS

Amides
AA Physical Status Class System
Carpule
Cartridge
Conscious sedation
Contraindication
Esters
Field block
General anesthesia
Infiltration
Local anesthesia
Lumen
Nerve block
Nitrous oxide
Pain
Paresthesia
Periodontal ligament injection
Topical anesthesia

FILL-IN QUESTIONS

1. Identify the length and gauge of the needle most commonly used to anesthetize each of the following teeth.

Tooth	Length	Gauge (ga)
a. #6	_____	
b. #10	_____	
c. #31	_____	
d. #20	_____	

2. Identify the parts of the syringe.

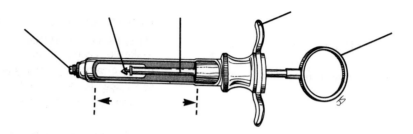

FIG. 23-1 Syringe.

a. _____

b. _____

c. _____

d. _____

e. _____

f. _____

3. Select the most common method of injection for each of the following situations.

Structure	Injection Method
a. Oral mucosa	_____
b. Maxillary teeth	_____
c. Mandibular anterior teeth	_____
d. A quadrant of mandibular teeth	_____

4. Explain in a step-by-step procedure the preparation of the syringe for an injection on tooth #30DO and the hidden transfer technique.

MATCHING QUESTIONS

Match the following terms with the definitions below.

_____ 5. Breech
_____ 6. 1½ inch needle
_____ 7. Nerve block
_____ 8. Thumb ring
_____ 9. Ampule
_____ 10. Protective sheath
_____ 11. 1-inch needle
_____ 12. Field block
_____ 13. Gauge
_____ 14. Carpule
_____ 15. Diaphragm

a. Part of syringe used to force anesthesia into tissue
b. May be used more than once
c. Area of syringe in which carpule is placed
d. Usually used in infiltration
e. Diameter of needle
f. Used once and then disposed
g. Usually used in nerve block
h. Same as carpule
i. Needle is attached to it
j. Cover over injection end of needle
k. Needle end of carpule
l. Commonly used on mandible
m. Commonly used on maxilla

MULTIPLE CHOICE QUESTIONS

16. Which of the following is a vasoconstrictor?
    1. Xylocaine
    2. Neo-cobefrin
    3. Carbocaine
    4. Epinephrine

    a. 1, 2, and 3
    b. 1 and 3
    c. 2 and 4
    d. 4 only
    e. All of the above

17. Which is the smallest gauge?
    a. 25
    b. 27
    c. 30

18. Which of the following is (are) characteristic of a local anesthetic?
    1. Patient remains conscious.
    2. Patient becomes unconscious.
    3. Selected regions of the body lose sensation.
    4. Sensation of the entire body is lost.
    5. Patient becomes semiconscious.

    a. 1, 2, and 4
    b. 1, 3, and 4
    c. 1 and 3
    d. 1
    e. 4

19. Which type of anesthetic provides anesthesia only to nerve endings located in the mucosa?
    a. Local
    b. Topical
    c. General

20. Which of the following methods of injection would provide anesthesia to an entire quadrant?
    a. Block
    b. Infiltration

21. Arrange the following steps in the proper sequence for a hidden syringe transfer. Number steps from 1 to 9.
    _____ a. Pass topical anesthetic.
    _____ b. Adjust operator's view of anesthetic solution.
    _____ c. Grasp operator's hand.
    _____ d. Place needle into protective covering with one hand.
    _____ e. Release operator's hand.
    _____ f. Pass 2- by 2-inch gauze to absorb blood or anesthetic solution.
    _____ g. Retrieve used syringe.
    _____ h. Pass syringe.
    _____ i. Pass 2- by 2-inch gauze to dry site.

CLINICAL APPLICATION

Make corrections in the following written narrative that are necessary to make the scenario accurate according to demonstration, reading, and lecture material, as well as consistent with OSHA standards.

The patient is to receive treatment on tooth #4. The patient's record indicates that because of his health history he is to have anesthesia without a vasoconstrictor. The assistant prepares the 1⅝-inch needle with Carbocaine with Neo-cobefrin. The aspirating syringe is assembled with the rubber plunger of the carpule inserted into the hub of the needle.

Before passing the syringe, the assistant passes the topical anesthetic for placement. When the syringe is passed to the operator, the protective cover is removed and accidently dropped on the floor.

The operator anesthetizes the site and passes the syringe to the assistant. The assistant lays the syringe in the preset tray cover and continues to pass instruments for the procedure.

CRITICAL-THINKING ACTIVITY

1. What steps can you take to ensure that the anesthetic syringe is properly prepared and ready for use in a treatment situation?

UNIT V

Basic Clinical Procedures

24 Oral Diagnosis

LEARNING OBJECTIVES

You will have mastered the material in this chapter when you can:

- Define the key terms
- Describe the process of oral diagnosis
- Describe the importance of a complete personal and medical history
- Explain the need to update a patient's personal and medical history
- Describe the procedure for obtaining vital signs
- Describe the use of consent forms, radiographs, laboratory studies, study models, and photographs in clinical evaluation
- List the data necessary for a complete dental clinical examination
- Describe an extraoral examination
- Describe an intraoral examination
- Identify common abbreviations and symbols used in charting a dental examination
- Explain the step-by-step procedure for obtaining diagnostic impressions
- Describe common laboratory reports
- Explain the development of a treatment plan
- Describe the process of case presentation

KEY WORDS

Adventitious
Blood pressure (BP)
Clinical examination
Clinical record
Dental history
Diagnosis
Diagnostic models
Diastole
Dyspnea
Hypertension
Hypotension
Hypothermia
Medical history
Occlusion
Patient history
Prognosis
Pyrexia
Sphygmomanometer
Stethoscope
Stridor
Systole
Temperature, pulse, and respiration (TPR)
Treatment plan
Vital signs

FILL-IN QUESTIONS

Describe the function of each of the following.

1. Patient registration and health history form:

2. Treatment record:

3. Initial examination form:

4. History update form:

5. Re-examination form:

6. Distinguish between personal, medical, and dental history. Identify at least five pieces of information which would be helpful in treating a patient that can be obtained from each of these forms of history.

Personal history

Medical history

Dental history

7. Explain why it is important to obtain a patient's vital signs before and at follow-up treatment.

8. Define the following vital signs, and answer the questions relating to each vital sign.

    a. TEMPERATURE

       Definition: _____

       1. What is a normal temperature?

       2. What factors would affect temperature?

       3. What effect would a raised temperature have on dental treatment?

4. Briefly describe how a temperature reading would be taken in a dental office.

5. At what other sites other than the mouth can a temperature reading be obtained?

    b. PULSE RATE

       Definition: _____

       1. What is a normal pulse rate?

       2. Describe fluctuations in pulse rate.

       3. In what locations can a pulse normally be obtained?

       4. Briefly describe the procedure for taking a pulse rate.

    c. RESPIRATION

       Definition: _____

       1. What is a normal respiration rate?

       2. Describe fluctuations in respiration rate.

       3. How is a respiration rate obtained?

       4. Briefly describe the procedure for obtaining a respiration rate.

d. BLOOD PRESSURE

Definition: _____

1. What is a normal blood pressure reading rate?

2. Under what conditions might a patient be referred for further evaluation of blood pressure to determine any abnormalities?

3. Define hypertension.

4. Define hypotension.

5. What are the potential health risks in the treatment of patients with either hypertension or hypotentions?

6. What is meant by *systole*?

7. What is meant by *diastole*?

9. State a blood pressure value that would indicate hypertension:

_____

State a blood pressure that would indicate hypotension:

_____

State a TPR value and a BP value that would indicate normal readings:

_____

10. Give the meaning for the following clinical abbreviations:

DM

AIDS

PA

REC

CNP

MATCHING QUESTIONS

Match each of the following with the instrument or device that is used to check it during an intraoral examination.

_____ 11. Interproximal caries
_____ 12. Furcation involvement
_____ 13. Periodontal depth
_____ 14. Tooth surface for caries

a. Explorer
b. Mirror
c. Ice pencil
d. Periodontal probe
e. Vitalometer
f. Bite-wing radiograph
g. Periapical radiograph

MULTIPLE-CHOICE QUESTIONS

15. To determine tooth vitality which of the following would *not* be used?
    1. Electronic pulp tester
    2. Ice pencil
    3. Percussion
    4. Mobility
    5. Heat
    6. Transillumination

    a. 1, 2, and 3
    b. 1, 2, 3, and 5
    c. 1, 2, 3, 4, and 5
    d. 4 only
    e. 6 only

16. Elements of informed consent include
    1. That consent be given freely
    2. That a description of treatment and diagnosis must be made in understandable language
    3. The right of the patient to ask questions and have them answered
    4. An explanation of the risks and benefits of the proposed treatment, estimate of success of treatment (prognosis) and alternative treatment plans

    a. 1 and 3
    b. 2 and 4
    c. 1, 2, and 3
    d. 1, 2, 3, 4, and 5
    e. 4 only

17. Which of the following would be considered implied consent?
    1. Use reasonable care in providing services in accordance with a set of community standards.
    2. Obtain an accurate health history for a patient before administering treatment.
    3. Employ competent personnel.
    4. Make provisions for complete emergency care in a timely manner.
    5. Explain the treatment, and obtain signed consent.

    a. 1, 3, and 5
    b. 1, 2, 3, and 4
    c. 2 and 4
    d. 5 only

18. When a patient health history is being reviewed, illnesses or conditions that might require alteration in medication or premedication for a routine prophylaxis might include
    1. Rheumatic fever
    2. Prolapsed valve
    3. Joint replacement
    4. Diabetes
    5. A prescription for coumadin

    a. 1, 2, and 5
    b. 1, 2, 3, and 5
    c. 1, 2, 3, 4, and 5
    d. 4 only

19. Inquiring about the drugs a patient is taking is necessary to
    1. Prevent potentially harmful drug interaction
    2. Develop an understanding of the total patient health profile
    3. Be aware of potential emotional or physical reactions during dental care
    4. Determine the need to interact with the patient's physician regarding patient care

    a. 1 and 3
    b. 2 and 4
    c. 1, 2, and 3
    d. 1, 2, 3, 4, and 5
    e. 1 only

20. Which of the following are components of an extraoral examination?
    1. Examination of the lips
    2. Measurement of the periodontal depth
    3. Facial symmetry
    4. Gait
    5. TMJ
    6. Color of the soft tissue

    a. 1 and 2
    b. 3 and 4
    c. 1, 3, 4, and 5
    d. 1, 2, 3, 5, and 6
    e. 1, 3, 4, 5, and 6

21. Which of the following are components of an intraoral examination?
    1. Status of frenum attachment
    2. Periodontal depth measurement
    3. Tooth mobility
    4. TMJ
    5. Examination of the teeth
    6. Color and texture of soft tissue

    a. 1, 2, and 3
    b. 1, 2, 3, and 5
    c. 2, 3, 5, and 6
    d. 1, 2, 3, 5, and 6
    e. 1, 2, 3, 4, 5, and 6

22. Which of the following are components of a thorough clinical examination?
    1. Photographs
    2. Laboratory studies
    3. Complete intraoral and extraoral examinations
    4. Radiographic findings
    5. Diagnostic findings
    6. Complete personal, dental and health histories

    a. 1, 2, and 3
    b. 1, 2, 3, 4, and 5
    c. 2, 3, 4, 5, and 6
    d. 1, 2, 3, 4, 5, and 6

23. A raised temperature is an indication of
    1. Infection
    2. Fatigue
    3. Exercise
    4. Korotkoff disease

    a. 1 and 3
    b. 2 and 4
    c. 1, 2, and 3
    d. 1, 3, and 4
    e. 4 only

24. If a patient is considered hypotensive, the blood pressure might be
    a. 80/120
    b. 110/52
    c. 210/104
    d. 132/80

25. If the assistant was unable to detect the systolic reading when taking a blood pressure reading, it would be wise to do the following:
    1. Have the patient remove any bulky clothing.
    2. Remove the air from the manometer.
    3. Reposition the stethoscope on the brachial artery.
    4. Place the patient in a different position.
    5. Ask a dentist to take the blood pressure reading.

    a. 1 and 3
    b. 2 and 4
    c. 1, 2, and 3
    d. 5 only

TRUE OR FALSE QUESTIONS

Place a **T** for True or an **F** for False to indicate whether each of the following statements is true or false.

_____ 26. Intraoral imaging illustrates to a patient precise oral detail in high detail with magnification.

_____ 27. Cosmetic imaging provides the patient with a "before-and-after" visual image of existing conditions, generating an image of what the tooth will look like when restored with various types of restorations.

_____ 28. When taking diagnostic impressions, the maxillary impression should be obtained first.

_____ 29. TPR and BP data should be obtained at every appointment.

_____ 30. Prognosis is the foretelling of the probable course of the disease.

_____ 31. Diagnosis and prognosis are synonymous terms.

_____ 32. When a patient has a history of hemophilia, it will be necessary to perform a biopsy before treatment.

_____ 33. It is necessary that each patient seen in the office have a baseline periodontal chart completed.

CLINICAL APPLICATION

Pair up with a peer in a treatment room and obtain TPRs and blood pressure readings from each other. Write each vital sign on a record, and have a third person obtain vital signs to verify that those you obtained are correct.

CRITICAL-THINKING ACTIVITIES

1. A new patient arrived for a dental appointment
    and you obtained the following vital signs:
    Temperature   100.4° F
    Respirations   60 breathes per min
    Pulse 72 beats per min
    Blood pressure 190/89

    Evaluate the vital signs, and identify what
    course of action might be taken at this point.

2. A new patient arrives for an appointment and
    completes the personal and health history
    profile. Contained within the profile are ques-
    tions regarding HIV. The patient has indicated
    a positive answer on the form. Would the
    dentist be responsible for providing this patient
    with required treatment? Explain your answer
    thoroughly.

25 Managing Emergency Needs of Patients

LEARNING OBJECTIVES

You will have mastered the material in this chapter when you can:

- Define the key terms
- Identify medical conditions or health changes that may affect a patient's dental treatment
- Explain the management of common dental emergencies
- Explain the management of common medical emergencies
- Describe the appropriate emergency equipment for a dental office
- Identify the ABCs of emergency care
- Describe the chain of command in a dental emergency
- Explain the procedure for CPR
- Describe the Heimlich maneuver

KEY TERMS

ABCs of emergency care
Abscess
Advanced cardiac life support (ACLS)
Anaphylactic shock
Avulsed tooth
Cardiopulmonary resuscitation (CPR)
Emergency medical service (EMS)
Epilepsy
Grand mal seizure
Heimlich maneuver
Hyperglycemia
Hypoglycemia
Jacksonian epilepsy
Petit mal seizure
Psychomotor seizure
Stoma
Syncope

FILL-IN QUESTIONS

1. What is considered an office emergency, and what major component is necessary to deal with an emergency?

2. The first step in the prevention of a medical emergency is to obtain a thorough patient history. Why is a patient history so important? Provide four reasons.

a. _____

b. _____

c. _____

d. _____

MATCHING QUESTIONS

Match each of the following terms with the correct definition:

_____ 3. Syncope
_____ 4. Petit mal
_____ 5. Stoma
_____ 6. CPR
_____ 7. ACLS
_____ 8. Prevention
_____ 9. Recognition

a. First step in preparing for an office emergency
b. Trendelenburg position is recommended for the patient who has this
c. Second step in preparing for an office emergency
d. The basics for reviving a patient
e. Form of epilepsy
f. Worst type of seizure for patient
g. Opening in throat for airway
h. Advanced level from the ABCs

MULTIPLE-CHOICE QUESTIONS

10. Training and readiness for medical emergencies is the primary responsibility of the
    a. Dentist
    b. Assistant
    c. Licensed assistant
    d. Office manager
    e. Hygienist

11. Patients who have a known history of cardiac disease should be given
    a. Morning appointments
    b. Afternoon appointments
    c. Appointments at the end of the day when other patients will not be in the office
    d. Appointments at any time

12. The site most commonly used in obtaining an accurate pulse rate in a patient is the
    a. Brachial artery
    b. Carotid artery
    c. Radial artery
    d. Temporal artery

13. Short dental appointments are often scheduled for patients with
    a. Allergies
    b. Herpetic lesions
    c. Cardiac problems
    d. Diabetes

14. A patient is seen for the purpose of having a crown seated, and it drops to the back of the throat. You should
    a. Give the patient water, and ask him or her to swallow.
    b. Have the patient sit up with head over knees.
    c. Allow the patient to cough the object out of his or her mouth.

15. The situation known as _____ is considered a compromised state of body functions and the means of assisting a patient with this condition is by placing the body in a position where the _____.
    1. Depression
    2. Shock
    3. Neurotic
    4. Head is flat and turned to the side
    5. Head is lower than the body
    6. Head and shoulders are higher than the rest of the body

a. 1 and 4
b. 2 and 5
c. 2 and 6
d. 3 and 5
e. 1 and 5

16. During a patient's epileptic seizure the dental team should make an effort to reduce the possibility of further injury by
    a. Holding the patient to prevent thrashing about
    b. Placing a padded object in the patient's mouth to prevent swallowing of the tongue
    c. Moving out of the area all objects that could cause injury to the patient during the seizure

17. When a patient is in need of CPR, chest compressions are performed by placing the heel of the hand
    a. Just above the heart
    b. Two to three finger widths above the inferior edge of the sternum
    c. Two to three finger widths above the superior edge of the sternum

18. The recommended course of care for a patient going into insulin shock is to
    a. Send the patient home to rest.
    b. Provide the patient with sugar or sweetened fruit drink.
    c. Administer an insulin injection.
    d. Provide the patient with protein.

19. If a patient has dry mouth with breath that smells of acetone, complains of thirst, and has a weak pulse, the most likely cause is
    a. Kidney stone attack
    b. Diabetic coma
    c. Hypertension
    d. Petit mal seizure

CLINICAL APPLICATION

1. A patient of record is seated for dental care, and you attempt to register the TPR and BP. The patient's BP is registered as 185/85, which is considerably higher than on past visits. What would you do at this point?

2. A mother calls about her young child who just fell off his skateboard and lost a front tooth. What would you direct the mother to do at this point. Be specific.

CRITICAL-THINKING ACTIVITY

A patient arrives in your office for an early-morning dental appointment before the dentist arrives. The patient complains to you about not feeling well, and about having clammy skin, racing pulse and slight numbness in the arm. What would you suspect as the possible problem? What would you do under these circumstances?

26 Preventive Dentistry

LEARNING OBJECTIVES

You will have mastered the material in this chapter when you can:

- Define the key terms
- Describe the factors relating to prevention in dentistry
- List common preventive procedures
- Describe motivation skills needed in patient education
- Define diet analysis
- Explain home care instructions for a variety of oral conditions
- Describe the techniques for the use of various oral hygiene devices
- Select appropriate toothbrush, floss, and auxiliary aids for patients with various needs
- Explain how an oral prophylaxis is a preventive procedure
- Describe the armamentarium and procedure for an oral prophylaxis
- Explain the function of fluoride and pit and fissure sealants as preventive agents
- List three types of topical fluoride, and explain how they are applied in an office setting
- List common types of self-administered topical and systemic fluorides
- Describe the armamentarium and procedure for applying topical fluorides and pit and fissure sealants.

KEY TERMS

Bass technique
Charters' technique
Dentrifice
Diet analysis
Disclosing agent
Flossing
Fluoride
Fones technique
Interdental aids
Modified Stillman's technique
Motivation
Oral hygiene aids
Oral hygiene score
Oral prophylaxis
Patient education
Pit and fissure sealants
Press-roll technique
Preventive dentistry
Scaler

FILL-IN QUESTIONS

1. Explain why the Food Guide Pyramid, rather than the Basic Four Food Groups, has become the standard guide for food consumption.

2. Using the information provided, chart the surfaces listed as disclosed plaque. After charting all 28 teeth, determine the percentage of tooth surfaces that have plaque accumulations.

   Plaque on tooth surfaces:

   #2^{M,D} #3^{D,B} #6^L #14^{D,B} #15^{M,B} #18^{D,L} #19^{M,L}
   #24^L #25^L #30^L

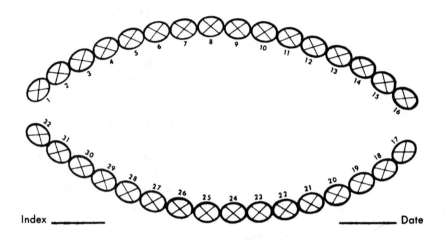

Index _____   _____ Date

FIG. 26-1 Plaque scoring chart.

3. What is the literal definition of a dental prophylaxis?

4. Name 3 substances that are removed from the teeth during an oral prophylaxis.

   a. _____

   b. _____

   c. _____

5. Name the three common forms of fluoride, and list an advantage and a disadvantage of each.

   Fluoride

   _____

   _____

   _____

   Advantage

   _____

   _____

   _____

   Disadvantage

   _____

   _____

   _____

6. List four goals of preventive dentistry.

   a. _____

   b. _____

   c. _____

   d. _____

MATCHING QUESTIONS

Match each of the terms listed below with the correct definition.

_____ 7. Sealants
_____ 8. Fluoride
_____ 9. Disclosing
_____ 10. Polishing
_____ 11. Flossing
_____ 12. Prophylaxis
_____ 13. Mouthguard
_____ 14. Curet scaler
_____ 15. Modified sickle scaler
_____ 16. Periodontal probe
_____ 17. Rubber cup

a. Used for coronal polishing
b. Removes calculus from all surfaces of teeth
c. Measures pocket depth
d. Removal of plaque, calculus, and stain
e. Identifies presence of plaque
f. Marks pocket depth
g. Removes plaque from the inter-area
h. Removing calculus f rom subgingival ar-eas of teeth
i. Removes deposits fr om posterior inter-proximal areas
j. Protects against oral injuries
k. Protects deep groove s in premolars and molar
l. Absorbed by all teeth
m. Removal of the ac-quired pellicle

Match each of the following recommended dental devices with a patient situation.

_____ 18. Super Floss™
_____ 19. Dentrifice with anodyne capability
_____ 20. Home fluoride rinse
_____ 21. Rubber-tipped stimulator
_____ 22. Floss holder
_____ 23. Bridge threader

a. Three-unit ce-mented prosthesis
b. Gingival swelling from mandibular anterior crowding
c. Gingival recession
d. Diastema
e. Removal of partial denture
f. Well water without fluoride
g. Arthritis

MULTIPLE-CHOICE QUESTIONS

24. What condition would be visible in the mouth of a patient who has excess fluoride in his or her system?
    a. Gray stains
    b. Mottled enamel
    c. Decalcification
    d. Mottled dentin

25. Plaque consists of
    a. Calculus
    b. Food debris
    c. Calcium bacteria
    d. Calcium and phosphate salts

26. The most effective caries reduction occurs with use of
    a. Topical fluoride
    b. Fluoridated water supply
    c. Fluoridated dentrifices

27. Which situation contraindicates the placement of pit and fissure sealants?
    a. Primary molars
    b. Decalcified teeth
    c. Moderately decayed teeth
    d. Deep fissures on posterior teeth
    e. Permanent premolars and molars

28. Plaque may be responsible for
    a. Only caries
    b. Stains
    c. Caries and periodontal disease
    d. Only periodontal disease
    e. Stains

29. The recommended fluoride concentration is
    a. 0.1 ppm
    b. 1 ppm
    b. 2 ppm
    c. 100 ppm

30. The following is true of disclosing a patient's mouth. It should
    1. Be done before brushing.
    2. Be done before and after brushing.
    3. Indicate areas of calculus.
    4. Indicate areas of plaque.
    5. Indicate areas of plaque and calculus.

    a. 1 and 3
    b. 2 and 4
    c. 2 and 3
    d. 2 and 5
    e. 1 and 5

CLINICAL APPLICATION

1. With a peer and a variety of oral hygiene devices, demonstrate and explain oral hygiene techniques as suggested in the textbook.

2. With a peer and fluoride materials, simulate a fluoride treatment.

CRITICAL-THINKING ACTIVITY

A 45-year-old female periodontal patient with heavy cervical plaque, a four-unit fixed bridge, and a mandibular denture needs instruction in proper home care. Answer the following questions as if you were providing instruction to the patient.

1. What method of toothbrushing and type of toothbrush would probably be recommended for this patient?

2. What auxiliary aids could you recommend, and for which areas would each be used?

UNIT VI

Restorative Procedures

27 Amalgam Restoration

LEARNING OBJECTIVES

You will have mastered the material in this chapter when you can:

- Define the key terms
- Describe the use of amalgam as a restorative material
- Review the G. V. Black cavity forms
- Describe the steps of a cavity preparation
- Identify and explain the phases of an amalgam procedure
- Identify the armamentarium and materials used in the amalgam restorative procedure
- Identify the parts and describe the assembly of a circumferential matrix band and retainer
- Describe the function of basic instruments used in the amalgam restorative procedure
- Explain procedural modifications in different amalgam procedures
- Explain the indications for a pin-retained amalgam, and identify the associated armamentarium

KEY TERMS

Anatomical carving
Caries removal
Convenience form
Extension for prevention
Opening phase
Outline form
Resistance form
Retention form
Smooth-surface carving

FILL-IN QUESTIONS

1. List an instrument, device or material that is commonly used for each of the following steps in a Class II amalgam procedure on tooth #30MO. Be thorough and specific in your answers.

   a. Checking for overhangs

   _____

   b. Interproximal carving

   _____

   c. Removal of gross amalgam

   _____

   d. Opening phase of preparation

   _____

   e. Final occlusal carving

   _____

   f. Planing walls of preparation

   _____

   g. Sealing dentin tubules

   _____

   h. Forming retention in preparation

   _____

   i. Final smoothing of cavosurface margin

   _____

   j. Smoothing and shaping matrix band

   _____

   k. Passing amalgam material to operator

   _____

   l. Condensing last increment of amalgam

   _____

   m. Placing zinc phosphate cement

   _____

n. Adapts band to tooth and creates interproximal space

_____

o. Shaping and forming cervical bevel

_____

p. Checking occlusion after final carving

_____

q. Outline form of preparation

_____

r. Remove excess caries manually

_____

s. Remove excess caries mechanically

_____

t. Forms missing wall for preparation during restorative phase

_____

u. Mixes amalgam

_____

2. Name the appropriate bur, the number and shank style. and the handpiece in which it would be placed to complete the following phases in cavity preparation.

a. Opening

_____

b. Outline

_____

c. Retention

_____

d. Caries removal

_____

3. State two purposes of wedge placement during a Class II amalgam restoration.

_____

_____

4. Identify the parts of the tofflemire retainer.

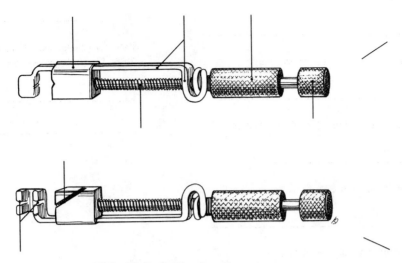

FIG. 27-2 Tofflemire diagram.

Occlusal aspect:

a. _____

b. _____

c. _____

d. _____

Gingival aspect:

e. _____

f. _____

5. Identify each of the items on the tray setup depicted below.

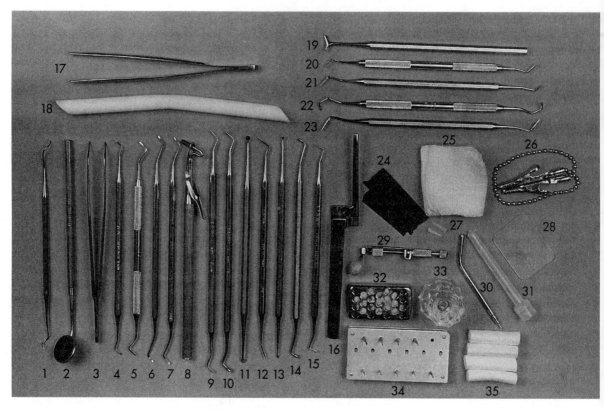

FIG. 27-2 Amalgam tray setup.

1. _____   14. _____

2. _____   15. _____

3. _____   16. _____

4. _____   17. _____

5. _____   18. _____

6. _____   19. _____

7. _____   20. _____

8. _____   21. _____

9. _____   22. _____

10. _____   23. _____

11. _____   24. _____

12. _____   25. _____

13. _____   26. _____

27. _____

28. _____

29. _____

30. _____

31. _____

32. _____

33. _____

34. _____

35. _____

6. Outline the duties that you as an assistant perform in each of the following categories.

   a. Anesthesia:

   b. Isolation:

   c. Cavity preparation:

   d. Cavity medication:

   e. Matrix band placement:

   f. Amalgam placement and condensation:

   g. Initial carving phase:

   h. Removal of matrix band and retainer:

   i. Final carving phase:

   j. Postoperative instructions:

MATCHING QUESTIONS

Match each of the following terms with the correct definition.

_____ 7. Wedge
_____ 8. Tofflemire retainer
_____ 9. Ivory retainer
_____ 10. Hollenback carver
_____ 11. Explorer
_____ 12. Mesial gingival marginal trimmer
_____ 13. Double spill
_____ 14. Class I
_____ 15. Class V
_____ 16. Hatchet

a. Removes unsupported enamel
b. Cervical caries
c. Separates teeth
d. Amalgam for a Class II preparation
e. Occlusal caries
f. Smooth-surface carving
g. Anatomic carving
h. Circumferential
i. Used to place bevels
j. Checks for caries
k. Amalgam for Class I preparation
l. Assists in restoring single proximal wall

MULTIPLE-CHOICE QUESTIONS

17. Which of the following techniques could be used for caries removal?
    1. No. 2 RA
    2. No. 1/4 FG
    3. Spoon excavator
    4. Enamel hatchet
    5. Explorer

    a. 1 and 2
    b. 1 and 3
    c. 2 and 4
    d. 1, 3, and 4
    e. 1, 3, and 5

18. Which of these cavity classifications would be candidates for an amalgam restoration?
    1. Class I
    2. Class II
    3. Class III
    4. Class IV
    5. Class V

    a. 1 and 2
    b. 2 and 3
    c. 3 and 4
    d. 1, 2, and 4
    e. 1, 2, and 5

TRUE OR FALSE QUESTIONS

Place a **T** for True or **F** for False as it refers to each of the following statements.

_____ 19. The matrix retainer and wedge are both placed from the buccal side.

_____ 20. The matrix retainer is placed on the lingual aspect, and the wedge is placed from the buccal aspect at the proximal surface involved.

_____ 21. The hatchet is used to remove unsupported enamel and soft carious debris.

_____ 22. The gingival marginal trimmer is used to place bevels on the proximal cervical floor and the pulpal floor.

_____ 23. Usually a single spill of amalgam will fill a Class I cavity preparation.

_____ 24. If it is necessary to mix additional amalgam spills during the filling of the preparation, all amalgam must be removed and new amalgam placed.

_____ 25. The bur most commonly used to create the resistance form is a No. 34 inverted cone.

_____ 26. A mesial and distal marginal trimmer is used during the completion of a Class II cavity preparation.

_____ 27. The ivory retainer is considered a circumferential matrix retainer.

_____ 28. A spirec drill is an instrument common to all pin procedures.

_____ 29. A No. 34 or No. 35 bur is preferred to make the initial pin-hold opening.

_____ 30. The autoclutch chuck contra angle is used in placing threaded pins.

_____ 31. Threaded pins must be precut with a wire cutter.

_____ 32. *Twist drill* and *spirec drill* are synonymous terms.

_____ 33. For compatibility with tooth structure, pins are commonly made of titanium and gold.

CLINICAL APPLICATION

Using the following form, select the instrument or device that would be used in each of the operative situations.

AMALGAM TRAY USAGE	2³	12⁵	14⁶	19MO	21DO	30^MO_D	32⁴
Anesthesia							
Long							
Short							
Rubber Dam							
Teeth isolated							
Clamp on							
Explorer							
Mirror							
Cotton pliers							
Spoon excavator							
Hatchet							
Mesial margin trimmer							
Distal margin trimmer							
Amalgam carrier							
#1 condensor							
#2 condensor							
Ward's C carver							
7 C							
5 C							
Ball burnisher							
Anatomical burnisher							
Matrix band							
Matrix retainer							
Wedges							
1.							
2.							
Dappen dish							
Cotton pellets							
Articulating paper							

CRITICAL-THINKING ACTIVITY

Identify errors in the following scenario, and make any corrections that are necessary to conform to standard operating procedures.

List the line number, the error, and the correction in the form below.

You are assisting a dentist at chairside for an amalgam procedure. The treatment room is decorated in pastel blues with navy carpet, and the patient compliments the dentist on the decor. The patient is having an amalgam placed on tooth #30^{MOD}. You prepare the anesthetic syringe with a 1-inch needle and a vasoconstrictor.

After anesthesia is administered, cotton rolls are placed in the patient's mandibular left quadrant. You provide the operator with a No. 6 round bur on the high-speed handpiece to open the preparation. You exchange the high speed handpiece with the low-speed handpiece with a No. ½ bur for placement of retentive grooves.

After the preparation is completed the operator indicates that she needs cavity varnish. You retrieve the cavity varnish from the mobile cabinet and pass a cotton pellet with the thumb forceps. A second application of varnish is needed, and you dip the pellet again and pass it for use.

The matrix band and retainer are prepared for the mandibular left quadrant before use, and they are passed at this time for placement. As the operator places the retainer, you prepare and pass a wedge for placement. The operator signals, and you mix a single spill of amalgam.

After the amalgam is mixed, the carrier is filled and passed. The large condenser is exchanged for the carrier and this procedure continues until most of the preparation is filled. As the preparation is almost filled, the operator requests the use of a small condenser.

The matrix band and retainer are removed and exchanged for the smooth-surface carver. The operator removes excess from the least accessible area, the proximal surface, first, and continues with anatomic carving. After the carving is completed, a full mouth rinse is administered and the patient is given post-operative instructions.

Error

Correction

28   Composite Restorations

LEARNING OBJECTIVES

You will have mastered the material in this chapter when you can:

- Define the key terms
- Describe the use of composite resin as a restorative material
- List the types of cavity preparations that are common with the use of composite resin as a restorative procedure
- Identify the steps of the composite resin restorative procedure
- Identify the armamentarium and materials used in the composite resin restorative procedure
- Describe the function of each instrument during the procedure

KEY TERMS

Bonding
Centrix syringe
Compules
Polymerize
Shade selection

FILL-IN QUESTIONS

1. Identify the basic steps in a Class III composite procedure.

   _____

   _____

   _____

   _____

   _____

   _____

   _____

   _____

2. Describe the advantages of light-cured restorative material as compared with chemically-cured restorative material.

   _____

   _____

   _____

3. Identify each of the items on the tray setup depicted below.

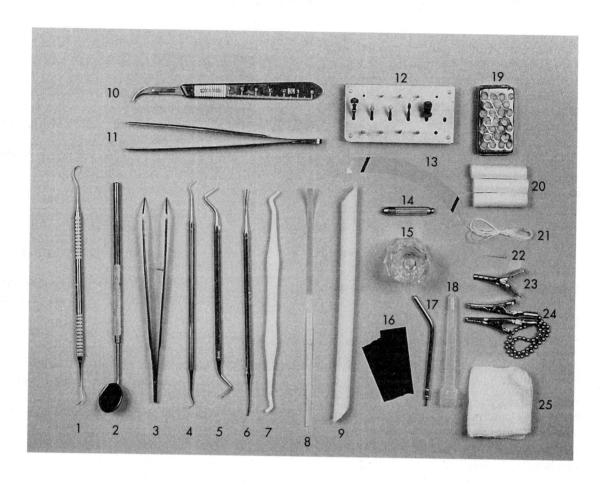

FIG. 28-1 Composite tray setup.

MULTIPLE-CHOICE QUESTIONS

4. Shade selection for an anterior esthetic restoration should be completed under which of the following conditions?
   1. With natural light and moist environment
   2. After cavity preparation and medication
   3. Before application of rubber dam
   4. To match the cervical portion of the tooth only
   5. Within the same oral environment as the tooth being restored

   a. 1 and 3
   b. 2 and 4
   c. 1, 2, and 3
   d. 1, 3, and 5

5. Which of the following would not be a form of matrix used for an anterior esthetic restoration?
   a. Celluloid strip
   b. Celluloid crown
   c. Tofflemire universal band

6. Which of the following instruments and materials are not necessary for a Class III composite restoration with ideal cavity depth?
   1. Cavity varnish
   2. Articulation paper
   3. Plastic instrument
   4. Cleoid-discoid carver
   5. Finishing strip
   6. Finishing disks and mandrel
   7. Cavitec
   8. White stones
   9. Rubber wheel
   10. Carbide burs

a. 1, 4, and 7
b. 1, 4, and 9
c. 2, 7, and 9
d. 4, 7, and 9

7. The hand instruments used to plane the walls and floors of the cavity preparation for a composite restoration might be
   1. Binangle chisel
   2. Cleoid-discoid carver
   3. Hoe
   4. Gingival marginal trimmer
   5. Wedelstaedt chisel

   a. 1 and 3
   b. 2 and 4
   c. 1, 3, and 5
   d. All of the above

8. When necessary, the preferred lining agent before insertion of a composite restoration is
   a. Calcium hydroxide
   b. Zinc oxide eugenol
   c. Cavity varnish
   d. Zinc phosphate

9. When the two-paste system is used for a composite material, the paste of one jar should not be cross-contaminated, for the following reason:
   a. It will cause the material to harden.
   b. It will prevent the material from hardening.
   c. The translucency will be diminished.
   d. Polymerization will be delayed.

10. After inserting, when can the final polish of light-cured composite be accomplished?
    a. Within 10 minutes
    b. Within 20 to 30 minutes
    c. After 8 hours
    d. As soon as polymerized

11. Which of the following statements are true regarding acid etching of enamel for a composite restoration?
    1. The acid etching agent forms a mechanical bond with the enamel.
    2. The acid etching is flooded onto the surface and rubbed vigorously.
    3. The material is applied with cotton pellets or small sponges that are supplied with the kit.
    4. The composite resin is placed before acid etching of enamel.

5. Acid etching is rinsed from the tooth after the recommended time, to stop the etching process.

   a. 1 and 3
   b. 2 and 4
   c. 1, 3, and 5
   d. 1, 2, 3, 4, and 5

12. When a composite restoration is being placed on a buccal one third of tooth #30, which of the following is the matrix of choice?
    a. Universal circumferential Tofflemire matrix
    b. Ivory noncircumferential matrix
    c. Class V composite matrix
    d. Celluloid strip

13. Which of the following statements are true regarding the acid etching process during placement of a composite restoration?
    1. In a Class III preparation a celluloid matrix is placed before etching to protect adjacent tooth enamel.
    2. After the bonding material is placed the surface is rinsed for 30 seconds.
    3. After etching the celluloid matrix is removed, and a new matrix is inserted before composite insertion.
    4. In a Class III preparation a celluloid matrix is not needed.

    a. 1 and 3
    b. 2 and 4
    c. 1, 2, and 3
    d. 4 only

TRUE OR FALSE QUESTIONS

Place a T for True or an F for False in the space provided as it refers to each statement.

_____ 14. Only light-cured composite restorative material may be placed in layers.
_____ 15. Composite restorative material may be placed in the anterior and posterior preparations.
_____ 16. When a celluloid crown form is being used during a composite procedure, a hole should be made in the incisal edge of the form.
_____ 17. Composite restorative material may be placed with an FP1 plastic instrument.

CLINICAL APPLICATION

With a peer and a manikin that has prepared teeth, simulate the treatment for a Class III composite procedure. Treat the simulation as if you had a live patient, using universal precautions and all the required steps in this procedure.

CRITICAL-THINKING ACTIVITY

A patient is seen in your office for a mesial incisal fracture that extended completely across the incisal edge of tooth #9. The patient was actively involved in the shade selection before placement. As the patient prepares to leave the treatment room, she complains to you about the color of the restoration.

What would you say to allay her concern? Is it necessary to remove the restoration and place a new one? Explain your answer.

29 Introduction to Prosthodontics

LEARNING OBJECTIVES

You will have mastered the material in this chapter when you can:

- Define the key terms
- Describe the scope and objectives of prosthetics
- Differentiate between the various types of fixed and removable dental prostheses
- Describe the function of various types of dental prostheses
- Describe the advantages and disadvantages of various types of fixed and removable prosthetic restorations
- Describe the preliminary steps to prosthetic treatment
- Explain the factors to be considered by the dentist when various prostheses are recommended to a patient
- Explain factors that are involved in becoming a successful prosthetic patient
- Explain the dental assistant's role in prosthetics

KEY TERMS

Abutment
Bilateral
Bridge
Cantilever bridge
Cosmetic imaging
Denture
Edentulous
Fixed prosthetics
Full-coverage crown
Implant
Inlay
Laminate
Maryland bridge
Obturator
Onlay
Overdenture
Pontic
Porcelain crown
Post and core
Prosthesis
Prosthetics
Removable prosthetics

Retainer
Surveying
Three-quarter crown
Tissue conditioning
Unilateral

FILL-IN QUESTIONS

1. Describe the difference between a fixed and a removable prosthesis. Be specific.
    Fixed:

    Removable:

2. From the diagrams below, identify and describe each of the restorations/prostheses.

    FIG. 29-1 Restorations/prostheses.

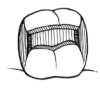

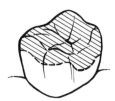 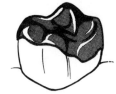

Cont'd.

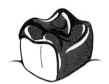

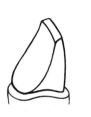
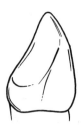

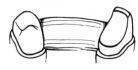
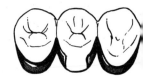

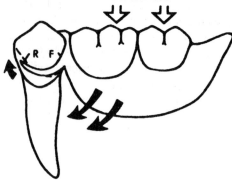

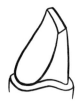
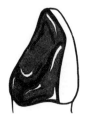

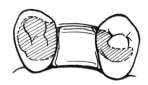
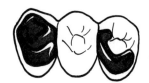

a.

b.

c.

d.

e.

f.

g.

h.

i.

3. Identify five potential dental anomalies that can occur from the loss of a single tooth.

a.

b.

c.

d.

e.

CRITICAL-THINKING ACTIVITIES

1. A patient of approximately 30 years of age is seen for an initial visit. After the patient is escorted to the treatment room, he mentions that he is interested in having the remaining teeth in his mouth extracted. Describe how you would educate this patient to the idea of keeping his teeth for a lifetime.

2. A 38-year-old female has lost the mandibular right second premolar. While she is in the office the dentist suggests that she have a fixed bridge. The dentist, who is short of time refers to her diagnostic models and suggests that she set up appointments for this treatment. She is unsure of the reasons for having this treatment and seems confused. She seeks your input about the reasons for replacing the single missing tooth. What do you suggest?

30 Fixed Prosthodontics

LEARNING OBJECTIVES

You will have mastered the material in this chapter when you can:

- Define the key terms
- Identify the purpose of the tooth preparations for fixed prosthetics
- Define the basic procedural sequence for the preparation, fabrication, and cementation of a fixed restoration
- Explain the role of the dental assistant in a fixed prosthetic procedure
- Describe common dental materials used in a fixed prosthetic procedure

KEY TERMS

Bite registration
Biologic principle
Burnishing
Cast
Cementation
Coping
Crucible former
Draw
Esthetic principle
Film thickness
Investing procedure
Ischemia
Laboratory prescription/requisition
Luxating
Mechanical principle
Occulusal clearance
Opposing model
Shade
Shimshock
Sprue
Surfactant
Tachycardia
Tissue retraction
Undercut
Wax elimination

FILL-IN QUESTIONS

1. Define the following terms, being thorough in your explanations.

   Bite registration:

   Draw:

   Final impression:

   Opposing impression:

   Occlusal clearance:

   Lost-wax technique:

   Margin finish:

   Gingival retraction:

2. What step(s) that is (are) used in an indirect gold technique is (are) eliminated during a direct gold technique?

3. What is meant by a loose or an open contact on a metal casting? How can this be corrected?

4. List the steps in a preparation appointment and a cementation appointment for a cast gold restoration.

Preparation

1.

2.

3.

4.

5.

6.

7.

8.

Cementation

1.

2.

3.

4.

5.

6.

7.

8.

5. Identify the instruments and devices on the preparation tray setup.

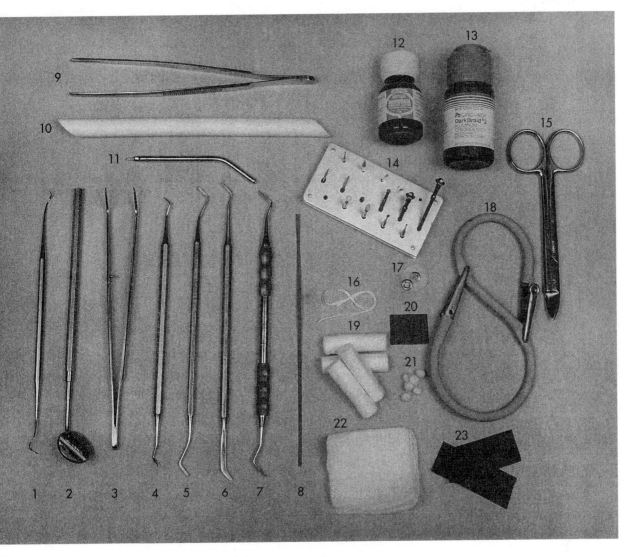

FIG. 30-1 Preparation tray setup.

6. Identify the instruments and devices on the cementation tray setup.

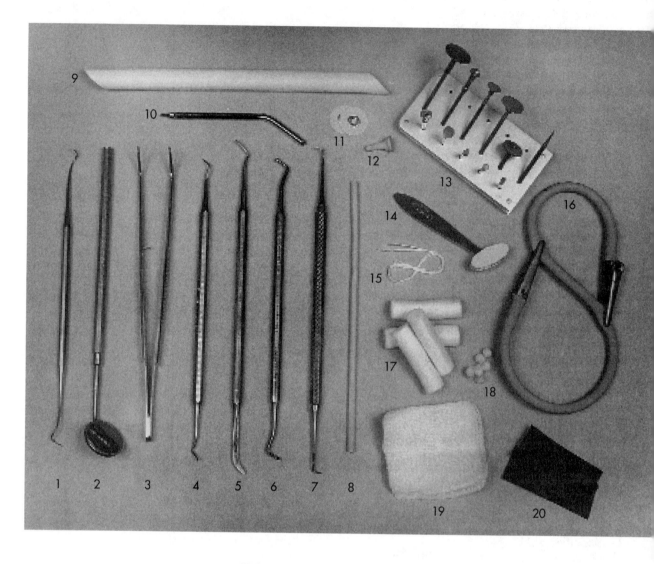

FIG. 30-2 Cementation tray setup.

MATCHING QUESTIONS

In the space provided, place the answer that best describes each term.

_____ 7. Maryland bridge
_____ 8. Class VI inlay
_____ 9. #8 FC
_____ 10. Missing #3 and #4
_____ 11. Laminate
_____ 12. Cantilever
_____ 13. Porcelain fused
　　　　 to metal crown

a. Requires minimal reduction of tooth structure on the facial surface
b. Support usually on one abutment only
c. Only three surfaces of the tooth are involved
d. Four-unit bridge required
e. Neck of metal usually seen at cervical line
f. Small dovetail retainers on abutment teeth
g. Candidate for porcelain crown
h. Only two surfaces of the tooth are involved

142

MULTIPLE-CHOICE QUESTIONS

14. To check occlusal clearance during a preparation for a gold crown you would
    a. Use baseplate wax.
    b. Use three thicknesses of 28-gauge green casting wax.
    c. Take an alginate impression.
    d. Test with the articulating paper.

15. Gingival retraction cord is placed
    a. Before the final impression
    b. After the final impression
    c. Usually during the preparation to define margins

16. When a crown preparation is being performed in a patient who has mitral valve dysfunction, and a sensitivity to epinephrine, which of the following would be used?
    1. Premedication
    2. Gingival retraction cord with clotting ability
    3. Anesthesia with a vasoconstrictor
    4. Anesthesia without a vasoconstrictor
    5. Nitrous oxide

    a. 1 and 3
    b. 1 and 4
    c. 1, 2, and 4
    d. 2, 4, and 5
    e. 5 only

17. Which of the following would *not* be used to remove a temporary restoration during a cementation procedure?
    a. Explorer
    b. Modified sickle scaler
    c. Spoon excavator
    d. Broken instrument with blunted end

18. After the patient has been anesthetized and the tooth to be prepared is isolated and prepared, the next steps are commonly to
    a. Check occlusal clearance, determine draw, take bite registration, place gingival retraction cord, take final impression, and temporize.
    b. Determine draw, check occlusal clearance, place gingival retraction cord, make temporary restoration, and take final impression.
    c. Check occlusal clearance, determine draw, place gingival retraction cord, take diagnostic impressions, and temporize.
    d. Check occlusal clearance, determine draw, place gingival retraction cord, take final impression, and temporize.

19. Which of the following restorations may be considered the abutments for a fixed bridge.
    1. Laminates
    2. Full gold crowns
    3. Porcelain veneer crowns
    4. Amalgam restorations
    5. Inlays

    a. 1, 2, and 3
    b. 2 and 5
    c. 2, 3, and 4
    d. 2, 3, and 5
    e. 1, 2, 3, and 5

20. The following steps are taken in the laboratory to process the impression and to create a full cast crown:
    a. Disinfect the impression, create the model, place separating medium, wax the pattern, invest the pattern, burnout, and casting
    b. Create the model, place separating medium, invest the pattern, wax and sprue the pattern, burnout, and casting
    c. Disinfect the impression, create the model, place separating medium, wax and sprue the pattern, invest, burnout, cast, and pickle the restoration

TRUE OR FALSE QUESTIONS

Place a T for True of an F for False in the space provided as it relates to each statement.

_____ 21. Zinc phosphate mixed to secondary consistency may be used for final cementation of a cast restoration.
_____ 22. To check occlusal clearance during a crown preparation for a patient, a specialized carbonized paper is used.
_____ 23. A die made from metal or stone is a positive reproduction of a tooth.
_____ 24. The pontic is the artificial tooth that replaces the missing natural tooth.
_____ 25. The patient may not need to be anesthetized during a gold cementation appointment.
_____ 26. The supports at the end of a bridge are called pontics.

_____ 27. Acrylic is placed in a tooth-colored crown to make a veneer crown for a temporary anterior tooth.

_____ 28. Gold solder is placed at the contact point to enlarge the area if the contact area is open during the try- in.

CLINICAL APPLICATION

Outline the steps in preparation for each type of restoration, and highlight steps that are eliminated or added in each procedure as it is compared to the others.

Class VI inlay

Full-coverage crown

Porcelain fused to metal crown

CRITICAL-THINKING ACTIVITY

A 75-year-old patient comes to your office for a consultation appointment to discuss his dental needs. The patient has been informed that he needs three bridges, maxillary right and left and mandibular right. He also explains that he has undergone periodontal surgery and treatment but has not gone back to the periodontist for 2 years. The following teeth have been extracted, #1, #2, #3, #5, #12, #13, #15, #16, #17, #24, #28, #29, #30, and #32. Is this patient a good candidate for extensive crown and bridge treatment? Explain your answer thoroughly.

31   <u>Removable Prosthodontics</u>

LEARNING OBJECTIVES

You will have mastered the material in this chapter when you can:

- Define the key terms
- Briefly describe the Kennedy classifications of removable prostheses
- Differentiate between the various types of removable prostheses
- Outline the typical appointment schedule for common removable prostheses
- Define the components of a removable prosthesis
- Describe the basic procedural steps necessary to create a removable prosthesis
- Describe home care for a removable prosthesis
- Define the various types of implants
- Describe the implant process

KEY TERMS

Adjustment
Alveolar ridge
Bar
Baseplate
Border molding
Centric relationship
Clasp
Complete denture
Connector
Conventional denture
Denture base
Diatoric hole
Duplicate denture
Endosteal
Face bow
Facing
Flask
Framework
Free way space
Immediate denture
Mortise
Mold
Muscle trimming
Occlusal rim
Osseointegration

Partial denture
Precision attachment
Rebase
Reline
Rest
Retentive area
Ridge
Saddle
Stippling
Subperiosteal
Tenon
Vertical dimension

FILL-IN QUESTIONS

1. List four problems that can be created by the loss of a single tooth.

   _____

   _____

   _____

   _____

2. Differentiate between what occurs at the delivery appointments for an immediate and a nonimmediate denture.

   _____

   _____

   _____

   _____

3. What occurs in a mouth that causes the following statement to be true "A denture does not last for a lifetime."

MATCHING QUESTIONS

In the space provided place the answer that best describes each term.

_____ 4. Border molding
_____ 5. Unilateral partial
_____ 6. Posterior palatal seal
_____ 7. Bilateral partial
_____ 8. Tenon
_____ 9. Mortise

a. First impressions with alginate for a denture patient
b. Both sides of mouth
c. Across the whole arch
d. Provides retention
e. Precision attachment
f. Add warm dental compound to the peripheries of the custom acrylic tray, and adapt the compound to the patient's muccobuccal and muccolabial folds
g. One side of the mouth
h. Female joint of precision attachment
i. Replaces the gingival tissue
j. Male joint of precision attachment

MULTIPLE-CHOICE QUESTIONS

10. Usually mandibular dentures are not as retentive as maxillary dentures, for the following reason:
    a. A mandibular denture covers less area as it replaces oral structures.
    b. The action of gravity tends to pull the maxillary denture loose.
    c. The mandibular ridge and the maxillary ridge are shaped differently.

11. A surveyor is used in partial denture construction to
    a. Assist in the attachment of wax rims for tooth placement
    b. Determine the position of the saddle
    c. Determine the placement of clasps

12. The segment of a partial denture that covers the ridge is known as the
    a. Lingual bar
    b. Clasp
    c. Saddle
    d. Major connector

13. The procedure known as flasking is necessary to
    a. Aid in placement of the teeth on the ridge
    b. Place wax rims
    c. Cure the acrylic
    d. Place all metal attachments

14. A denture reline is necessary to
    a. Place new denture teeth on old frame
    b. Create a different facial contour
    c. Adapt the denture to tissue contour

TRUE OR FALSE QUESTIONS

Place a **T** for True and an **F** for False in the space provided as it relates to each statement.

_____ 15. When teeth for a removable prosthesis are selected, the shape of a patient's face contributes to the selection of a mould.
_____ 16. A person's complexion relate to selection of shade of teeth for a prosthesis.
_____ 17. The objective of border molding is to replicate the border of the denture while tissues are being manipulated or are actively moving.
_____ 18. Gutta-percha is placed on the peripheral border of a tray during border molding.
_____ 19. _Clasp_ and _rest_ are synonymous terms.
_____ 20. _Immediate_ and _conventional_ dentures are synonymous terms.
_____ 21. The loss of a single tooth in an arch can be the initial stage in becoming a dental cripple.
_____ 22. The lingual bar on a maxillary denture is a major connector.
_____ 23. The palatal bar on a maxillary denture is a minor connector.
_____ 24. An extension from the lingual bar to a clasp or rest would be a minor connector.
_____ 25. Stippling is done on the internal portion of a denture.
_____ 26. Capillary-like fibers can be imbedded in a denture base to recreate a lifelike appearance of oral mucosa.

CLINICAL APPLICATION

A patient has recently had the posterior teeth on the maxillary arch removed in preparation for a full denture, and the anterior teeth are retained. Explain the following.

What type of denture is the patient likely to have?

About how long will it be before the first appointment in denture construction will take place after surgery?

State at least two reasons for retaining the anterior teeth.

The patient has returned to the office after the appropriate time for posterior tissue healing. Explain the sequence of appointments, making a brief statement about what will be done at each appointment until the denture is inserted. What type of follow-up appointments will this patient need?

CRITICAL-THINKING ACTIVITY

You are with a friend who has complete dentures and you notice the conditions listed below. Provide a possible explanation for why each situation may occur.

1. The person's profile is wrinkled around the lips.

2. There is a clanking sound of the denture when the patient speaks.

3. The person cannot hold her lips together.

32 Temporary Restorations

LEARNING OBJECTIVES

You will have mastered the material in this chapter when you can:

- Define the key terms
- Identify the difference between intracoronal and extracoronal temporary restorations
- Explain the functions of a temporary restoration
- Describe the procedure for the construction of temporary restorations
- Describe the procedure for the placement of all temporary restorations
- Identify the criteria for a clinically acceptable temporary restoration

KEY TERMS

Acrylic crown
Aluminum crown
Coping
Extracoronal dressing
Festoon
Interim dressing
Intracoronal dressing
Stainless steel crown
Temporary restoration

FILL-IN QUESTIONS

1. List the common reasons for placing a temporary restoration during the interim between preparation and cementation appointments.

   _____

   _____

   _____

   _____

   _____

2. What type of temporary restoration could be used for the teeth involved in each of the following situations?

   a. #3 to #5 bridge _____

   _____

   b. #8 porcelain veneer crown _____

   _____

   c. #19^{MOD} inlay _____

   _____

   d. #28 porcelain veneer crown _____

   _____

   e. #31 full coverage crown _____

   _____

MULTIPLE-CHOICE QUESTIONS

3. The primary functions of a temporary restoration are to
   1. Avoid hypereruption
   2. Avoid mesial drift
   3. Protect the teeth from sensitivity
   4. Improve esthetics
   5. Improve mastication

   a. 1 and 2
   b. 2, 3, and 4
   c. 2, 3, 4, and 5
   d. All of the above

4. Which of the following could be used as a temporary restoration for a posterior tooth that has been prepared for a full crown?
   1. Aluminum crown with acrylic wash
   2. Celluloid crown form with zinc phosphate cement
   3. Custom-made acrylic crown
   4. Intracoronal ZOE
   5. Preformed aluminum crown

   a. 1 and 2
   b. 1 and 3
   c. 1, 3, and 4
   d. 1, 3, and 5

5. Trimming of the temporary crown margins to fit the prepared tooth is called
   a. Burnishing
   b. Border molding
   c. Festooning
   d. Crimping
   e. Contouring

6. On a properly trimmed temporary crown, the margins should fit the prepared tooth
   a. Subgingivally
   b. Supragingivally
   c. At or 1 mm short of the crown margins
   d. At or 1 mm beyond the crown margins

7. Complete removal of a temporary restoration from an inlay preparation is essential because the
   a. Cement will irritate the pulp.
   b. Inlay will not seat completely.
   c. Remaining cement will interfere with the set of the final cement.
   d. Remaining cement will destroy the cavity varnish.

8. Which of the following cements would be most appropriate for use when cementing a temporary crown?
   1. ZOE
   2. Glass ionomer
   3. Zinc phosphate
   4. Low-strength luting agent
   5. Zinc polycarboxylate

   a. 1 and 4
   b. 1, 2, and 5
   c. 1, 3, and 5
   d. all of the above

9. The advantages of using an acrylic wash in an aluminum temporary crown include the following:
   1. The wash provides an anodyne effect.
   2. Increased strength is provided.
   3. Easier removal is provided.
   4. Better retention is provided.
   5. The wash increases wear resistance.

   a. 1, 2, and 4
   b. 1, 3, and 5
   c. 2, 3, and 4
   d. 2, 4, and 5

10. Which of the following would be appropriate as temporary restoration on an anterior crown preparation?
    1. ZOE cement
    2. Celluloid crown form
    3. Polycarbonate crown form
    4. Aluminum preformed crown
    5. Custom-made acrylic crown

    a. 1 and 2
    b. 1 and 3
    c. 2 and 5
    d. 2, 3, and 5

11. Which of the following cements is ideal as an intracoronal temporary restoration?
    a. Zinc polycarboxylate
    b. Glass ionomer
    c. Zinc phosphate
    d. Zinc oxide eugenol

12. Intracoronal temporary restorations can be inserted on which of the following preparations?
    1. Class I
    2. Class II
    3. Class III
    4. Class V
    5. Class VI (modified Class II)

    a. 2 and 5
    b. 1, 2, and 5
    c. 1, 3, 4, and 5
    d. All of the above

13. Which of the following describes clinically acceptable marginal ridges of an intracoronal temporary crown? They should
    1. Be cervical to the contact area
    2. Be at the same height as the adjacent tooth
    3. Be coronal to the contact area
    4. Follow the buccal and lingual contours of the tooth
    5. Be slightly higher than the adjacent tooth

    a. 2 and 4
    b. 1, 2, and 4
    c. 2, 3, and 4
    d. 2, 3, 4, and 5

14. If a properly trimmed aluminum crown flairs out at the cervical margin, you should do the following:
    1. Retrim the margins.
    2. Force the margins in with an explorer.
    3. Cement and then contour the crown after the cement is set.
    4. Use contouring pliers.
    5. Check the margins with an explorer.

    a. 2 and 3
    b. 1 and 5
    c. 4 and 5
    d. 1, 4, and 5

CLINICAL APPLICATION

1. Obtain a model with prepared teeth that require the placement of a temporary restoration. Create temporary restorations for intracoronal and full crown preparations. Follow the guidelines for clinically acceptable restorations as outlined in Chapter 32 of Comprehensive Dental Assisting: A Clinical Approach.

   After completing them, have the temporary restorations evaluated for clinical acceptance. Continue fabricating temporary restorations until each task is mastered.

CRITICAL-THINKING ACTIVITY

Describe the suggestions you would make to a patient in the following circumstances:

A patient who was seen a week ago for a crown preparation and temporization of tooth #30 calls to complain that the temporary crown has fallen off the tooth. The patient is leaving town tomorrow and wants to cancel the cementation appointment scheduled for next week and come in the week after that. What should your suggestions to this patient be?

UNIT VII

Specialized Procedures

Part Eight

Specialized Procedures

33 Endodontics

LEARNING OBJECTIVES

You will have mastered the material in this chapter when you can:

- Define the key terms
- Describe the scope of endodontics
- Describe the symptoms and etiology of an endodontically involved tooth
- Identify diagnostic tests used in endodontics
- Explain the importance of radiography in endodontics
- Identify and explain the function of specialized endodontic armamentarium
- Describe the physical characteristics and function of common intracanal instruments
- Identify the use of common intracanal medications
- Describe the basic procedures common to an endodontic practice
- Describe surgical procedures commonly found in endodontics
- Explain the function and process of vital and nonvital bleaching
- Identify the role of the dental assistant in various phases of endodontic treatment

KEY TERMS

Abscess
Actinomycosis
Apexification
Apexogenesis
Apical periodontitis
Apicoectomy
Bacteremia
Bicuspidization
Biomechanical cleansing
Bleaching
Broach
Buccal object rule
Cellulitis
Endodontic file
Extirpation
Fistula
Hemisection
Hyperemia

Master cone
Necrosis
Obturation
Osteomyelitis
Periapical abscess
Periodontal involvement
Pulpectomy
Pulpitis
Pulpotomy
Pulp stone
Reamer
Replant

FILL-IN QUESTIONS

1. When a solution such as sodium hypochlorite is used in a canal during biomechanical cleansing, what are its functions?

   a. _____

   b. _____

   c. _____

2. Identify five common diagnostic tools that are used in endodontics.

   a. _____

   b. _____

   c. _____

   d. _____

   e. _____

3. Identify four situations in which endodontic therapy is warranted.

   a. _____

   b. _____

   c. _____

d. _____

4. Explain what is meant by each of the following:

    a. Vertical pressure and lateral condensation:

    b. Never rotate a Hedstrom file:

    c. Never skip a file size:

5. What is the function of each of the following devices that are used in an endodontic procedure?

    a. Paper points:

    b. Sterile glass slab:

    c. Electric vitalometer:

    d. Spreader:

    e. Round bur:

    f. Rubber or metal stops:

    g. Temporary stopping:

    h. Zinc phosphate cement:

    i. Irrigating syringe:

    j. Broach:

    k. File:

    l. Cotton roll:

    m. Endodontic ruler:

    n, Orifice bur:

    o. Rubber dam:

    p. Final-point radiograph:

    q. Trial-point length:

6. Define and describe the procedure for each of the following:

    a. Vital bleaching:

    b. Hemisection:

    c. Pulpotomy:

d. Pulpectomy:

e. Apicoectomy:

MULTIPLE-CHOICE QUESTIONS

7. Gutta-percha material is used
   1. As a temporary stopping
   2. To irrigate the root canal
   3. To fill the filed canal
   4. As a trial point
   5. As a final point

   a. 1 and 3
   b. 1 and 4
   c. 3 and 5
   d. 1, 2, and 3

8. Endodontic files are used as to
   a. Gain access to the canal
   b. Enlarge the root canal
   c. Drain an infected canal

9. Obtaining an accurate measurement of the root canal length is necessary to
   a. Extend the final point 1 mm past the apex
   b. Obtain a sterile root canal
   c. Avoid creating periapical irritation near the apex

10. A vitalometer reading of 9 to 10 indicates that the tooth is
    a. Within normal ranges
    b. Nonvital
    c. Pyrexic
    d. Near death

TRUE OR FALSE QUESTIONS

Place a **T** for True or an **F** for False in the space provided next to each statement.

_____ 11. A Young's frame is radiolucent.
_____ 12. CMCP is used during biomechanical cleansing.
_____ 13. Gutta-percha cones are the usual final fill material.

_____ 14. An apicoectomy provides for an opening through the coronal portion of the tooth to control infection.
_____ 15. A trial-point radiograph is taken of the master cone to ensure that the cone fits 1.0 mm beyond the apical stop.
_____ 16. A barbed broach is used to enlarge a canal during biomechanical preparation.
_____ 17. The master gutta-percha cone is seated during final filling, before placement of supplemental gutta- percha points.
_____ 18. A cotton pellet saturated with CMCP, formocresol, or sodium hypochlorite is placed during the interim appointment.
_____ 19. A Hedstrom file is the most abrasive of the intracanal instruments.

CRITICAL-THINKING ACTIVITY

Explain why it is important to save a tooth by means of endodontic therapy.

34 Oral and Maxillofacial Surgery

LEARNING OBJECTIVES

You will have mastered the material in this chapter when you can:

- Define the key terms
- Describe the role of the oral surgery assistant
- List differences in design between an oral surgery and a general dental office
- Identify common medical conditions that can affect dental treatment
- Identify various types of antianxiety techniques and describe the advantages and disadvantages of each
- Name and describe the function of the types of instruments normally found on an oral surgery tray
- Describe the steps in tooth extraction
  Describe other common oral surgical procedures
- Explain common postoperative instructions for an oral surgery patient
- Discuss the role of the hospital in operative dentistry and maxillofacial surgery procedures

KEY TERMS

Anesthesiologist
Biopsy
Chisel
Conscious sedation
Electrocardiogram (EKG)
Elevator
Endotracheal tube
Extraction
Exodontia
Exfoliative cytology
Forceps
Frenectomy
Intravenous (IV)
Nitrous oxide
Orthognathic surgery
Periosteal elevator
Oximeter
Rongeur forceps
Stent
Surgical curette
Surgical dressing
Surgical suction tip
Suture
Trendelenburg
Titrate

FILL-IN QUESTIONS

1. List four major areas of treatment for an oral surgeon.

    a. _____

    b. _____

    c. _____

    d. _____

2. List three minor areas of treatment for an oral surgeon.

    a. _____

    b. _____

    c. _____

3. Identify and list four common postoperative instructions for patients after an extraction.

    a. _____

    b. _____

    c. _____

    d. _____

4. Name five common postoperative complications or complaints that might occur.

    a. _____

    b. _____

    c. _____

159

d. _____

e. _____

5. Identify the following instruments:

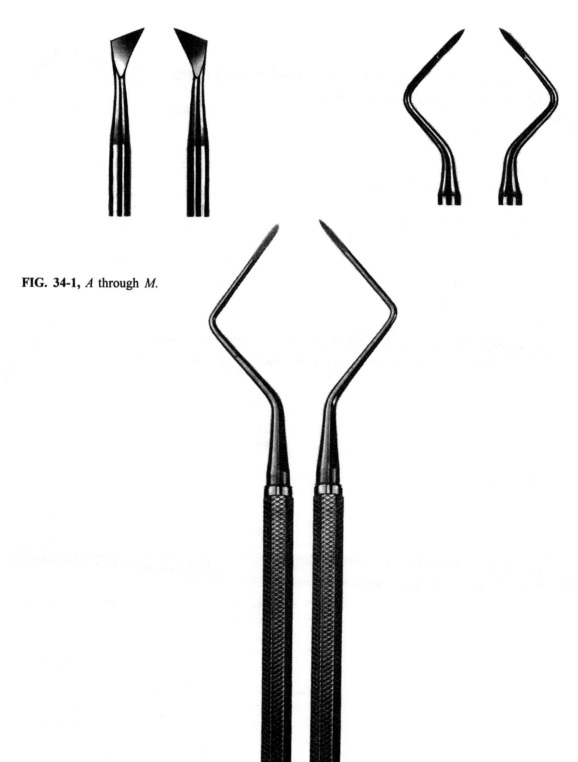

FIG. 34-1, *A* through *M*.

Cont'd.

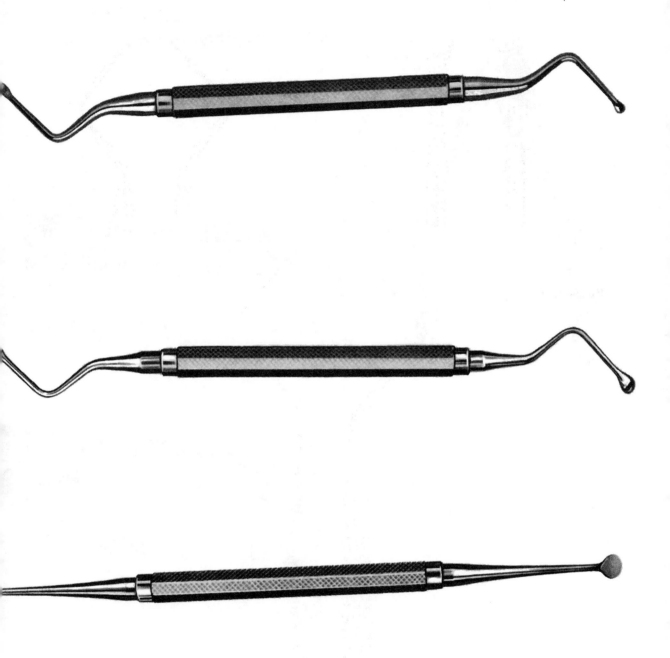

Cont'd.

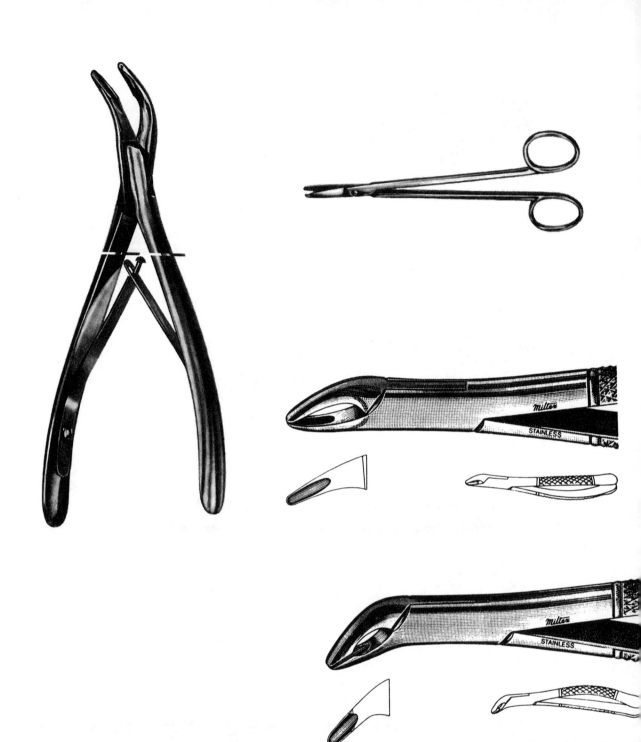

Cont'd.

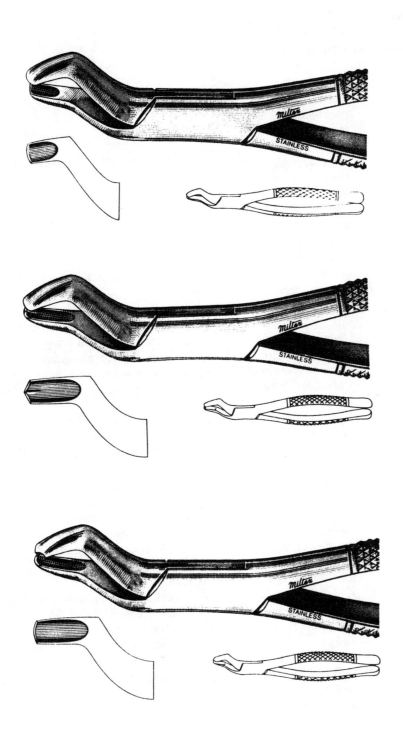

MATCHING QUESTIONS

Match the terms listed below with the descriptions on the right.

_____ 6. Periosteal elevator

_____ 7. Scalpel

_____ 8. Elevator

_____ 9. Ronguers

_____ 10. Curette

_____ 11. Cowhorn forceps

_____ 12. 151S forcep

_____ 13. 88R forcep

_____ 14. 150 forcep

_____ 15. Root tip pick

a. Universal forcep used for deciduous mandibular teeth

b. DE instrument designed with a broad or narrow rounded bevel on each end for lifting and turning back a flap of tissue and periosteum

c. A small, delicate, straight-bladed or contra angle-bladed instrument used for the removal of root tips

d. Universal lower forcep used for first and second molars when roots are not fused

e. A scissor type of surgical instrument that has cutting edge on the tips of beaks for bone contouring

f. A delicate surgical knife handle designed to receive interchangeable blades

g. Universal upper forcep used for anteriors and premolars

h. Placed interproximally to loosen teeth before forceps are used

i. DE instrument with spoon-shaped blade ends that is used for cutting epithelial attachment and debridement

j. Maxillary molar forcep with three beaks designed to fit configuration of maxillary molar roots

MULTIPLE-CHOICE QUESTIONS

16. What is the most common method of instrument transfer during an oral surgery procedure?
    a. One-handed pen grasp
    b. Two-handed pen grasp
    c. One-handed palm grasp
    d. Two-handed palm grasp

17. A common form of local anesthetic used in oral surgery procedures would be one
    a. With a vasoconstrictor, of slow onset and of long duration
    b. With a vasoconstrictor, of rapid onset and of short duration
    c. Without a vasoconstrictor, of rapid onset and of short duration
    d. Without a vasoconstrictor, of slow onset and of long duration

18. Patient monitoring during intravenous sedation is the responsibility of the
    a. Dental assistant
    b. Dentist
    c. Dental team
    d. Surgical dental assistant

19. The following instrument is commonly used to debride the tooth socket:
    a. Rongeur
    b. Surgical curette
    c. Root tip pick
    d. Elevator

20. In a surgical procedures nitrous oxide is used primarily as a(n)
    a. Inhalation gas, to enable the patient to breath easier
    b. Local anesthesia
    c. Inhalation sedative gas to render the patient unconscious
    d. Inhalation sedative agent

CRITICAL-THINKING ACTIVITY

Compare the following types of biopsy, and explain the differences and the reasons for performing each type:

Excisional:

Incisional:

Exfoliative:

Cytologic:

Exploratory:

35 Orthodontics

LEARNING OBJECTIVES

You will have mastered the material in this chapter when you can:

- Define the key terms
- Identify and classify the different types of malocclusion
- Describe the dental discrepancies that may be present in a malocclusion
- Identify the possible causes of malocclusion
- Differentiate between interceptive and corrective phases of orthodontic treatment
- Describe the types of diagnostic records used in orthodontic treatment planning
- Differentiate between removable and fixed appliances
- Identify the components of the fixed appliance system
- Describe the biologic mechanism of tooth movement
- Identify the basic orthodontic instruments and their use in placement of the appliances

KEY TERMS

Angle's classification of malocclusion
Archwire
Bracket
Class I
Class II
Class III
Corrective treatment
Crossbite
Elastics
Fixed appliance
Headgear
Interceptive treatment
Ligature tie
Malocclusion
Orthodontic band
Overbite
Overjet
Prognathic
Removable appliance
Retrognathic
Separator

FILL-IN QUESTIONS

1. Identify four components of an orthodontic record.

    a. _____

    b. _____

    c. _____

    d. _____

2. Describe the following items as they apply to orthodontics.

    a. Rubber bands:

    b. Frankel appliance:

    c. Bionator appliance:

    d. Herbst appliance:

3. A patient in an orthodontic practice is to have bands seated and orthodontic treatment begun. Explain the step-by-step procedure for selecting the bands, seating them on posterior teeth, and through the process of attaching brackets on the anterior teeth. In this discussion list the instruments commonly used for this procedure.

MULTIPLE-CHOICE QUESTIONS

4. Environmental factors that cause malocclusion may be all *except* which of the following?
   a. Large teeth
   b. Thumb sucking
   c. Abnormal swallowing
   d. Mouth breathing

5. The Angle's classification of occlusal relationships is based primarily on the
   a. Presence of crossbites
   b. Size of the overjet
   c. Number of rotated teeth
   d. Relationship of the maxillary first molar with the mandibular first molar

6. Which of the following statements about an open bite is false?
   a. It is often associated with a thumb or finger habit.
   b. It is often associated with a tongue thrust.
   c. It is the opposite of an impinging overbite
   d. It is most frequently found in the buccal segments.

7. Which of the following describes an Angle's classification of class II, division 2?
   1. Maxillary incisors in linguoversion
   2. Maxillary incisors in labioversion
   3. Mandibular first molars in distal relationship to maxillary first molars
   4. Mandibular first molars in mesial relationship to maxillary first molars
   5. Mesiobuccal cusp of maxillary first molar in mesiobuccal groove of mandibular first molars

   a. 1 and 3
   b. 2 and 3
   c. 2 and 4
   d. 2 and 5

8. Which of the following describe an Angle's classification of class II, division 1?
   1. Maxillary incisors in linguoversion
   2. Maxillary incisors in labioversion
   3. Mandibular first molars in distal relationship to maxillary first molars
   4. Mandibular first molars in mesial relationship to maxillary first molars
   5. Mesiobuccal cusp of maxillary first molar in mesiobuccal groove of mandibular first molar

   a. 1 and 3
   b. 2 and 3
   c. 2 and 4
   d. 2 and 5

9. Which of the following statements are true as they relate to elastic posterior separators?
   1. The separators are placed to create temporary space between teeth, allowing room for bands.
   2. Separator must completely surround contact area.
   3. elastic separating pliers are used for placement.
   4. Separators, like dental floss, are stretched and "see-sawed" through the contacts.
   5. The number of separators that are placed is noted on patient's record.

   a. 1, 2, and 3
   b. 3 and 4
   c. 1, 2, 3, and 4
   d. 1, 2, 3, 4, and 5

10. When orthodontic bands are being sized for mandibular premolars and molars, the band is first seated on the _____ aspect.
    a. Buccal
    b. Lingual
    c. Mesial
    d. Distal

11. Which of the following statements are true for sizing orthodontic bands?
    1. The gingival edge of the band goes over the tooth first.
    2. The occlusal edge of the band goes over the tooth first.
    3. A mallet and band driver may be used in seating the band.
    4. Bands are preformed stainless steel rings.
    5. Band sizes are universal, and bands can be adapted to fit any tooth.

    a. 1 and 3
    b. 1, 3, and 4
    c. 1, 3, and 5
    d. 2, 3, and 4

12. Ligature wires are secured in place by
    a. Bonding
    b. Means of elastic separators
    c. Cementing with zinc phosphate
    d. Twisting them to a length of 4 to 5 mm

13. Which of the following describes (describe) a class III malocclusion?
    1. Mandibular first molar is retruded in relationship to the maxillary first molar.
    2. Mandibular first molar is protruded in relationship to the maxillary first molar.
    3. Mesiobuccal cusp of the maxillary first molar is in the mesiobuccal groove of the mandibular first molar.
    4. Convex facial profile
    5. Concave facial profile

    a. 2 only
    b. 1 and 4
    c. 2 and 5
    d. 3 and 5

14. Which of the following statements is *not* true regarding toothbrushing in orthodontic patients?
    a. Patient must concentrate on the area between the band the gingival tissue.
    b. Bands and wires will become dull and tarnished from the oral fluids, which is not indicative of poor toothbrushing.
    c. Teeth that are blocked out and rotated require special attention when brushing.
    d. If a patient is unable to brush after eating, he or she should rinse vigorously with water.

CLINICAL APPLICATION

Using universal precautions in a prepared clinic setting, take turns completing orthodontic examinations on several peers. During each examination evaluate the individual for the presence of open bite, over bite, Angle's classification of malocclusion, rotated teeth and other orthodontic anomalies. After each examination have your instructor or employer check the accuracy of your examination.

CRITICAL-THINKING ACTIVITY

A patient is evaluated in the office and the dentist suggests that the patient needs to have extensive orthodontic treatment. There appears to be a severe crossbite on both sides of the arch. The child seems excited about the potential to improve her appearance and seems anxious to have treatment.

The mother says she had a lot of problems, too, but outgrew them, and she thinks the child should just grow up and see how things turn out. What might a dentist discuss with this patient?

36 Pediatric Dentistry

LEARNING OBJECTIVES

You will have mastered the material in this chapter when you can:

- Define the key terms
- Define the specialty of pediatric dentistry
- Describe the scope of pediatric dentistry
- Explain the role of the dental assistant in pediatric dentistry
- Describe common behavior patterns or stages in children
- Describe behavior management of children in the dental office
- Identify common treatment procedures in pediatric dentistry
- Identify urgent care treatment in pediatric dentistry
- List the signs and symptoms of child abuse
- Identify materials and equipment unique to pediatric dentistry

KEY TERMS

Behavior management techniques
Behavior patterns
Flooding
Hand-over-mouth (HOM)
Modeling
Papoose board
Pediatric dentistry
Show-and-tell
Validation

FILL-IN QUESTIONS

1. Are children little adults? Explain your answer.

2. Identify five tasks that the dental assistant may perform in a pediatric practice.

   _____

   _____

   _____

   _____

   _____

3. List five manifestations which could be observed during a clinical examination that might be seen in an abused child.

   _____

   _____

   _____

   _____

   _____

MULTIPLE-CHOICE QUESTIONS

4. Which of the following is *not* considered a behavior management technique for dealing with the child patient?
   a. Hand-over-mouth
   b. Flooding
   c. Modeling
   d. All of the above

5. Types of dental treatment commonly performed in the pediatric patient include the following:
   1. Pit and fissure sealants
   2. Prophylaxis
   3. Full cast crowns
   4. Stainless steel crowns
   5. Amalgam restorations

   a. 1, 2, and 3
   b. 2, 4, and 5
   c. 1, 2, 4, and 5
   d. All of the above

TRUE OR FALSE QUESTIONS

Place a **T** for True or an **F** for False in the space provided next to each statement.

_____ 6. Drug therapy as a behavior management technique is the most accepted course of action for treatment of the child patient.

_____ 7. Stainless steel crowns are placed as a protective crown in the mouth of a pediatric patient.

_____ 8. If a child is not behaving appropriately during dental treatment, it is advisable to bring the parent or caregiver into the treatment room.

_____ 9. A pulpectomy is commonly performed on teeth of a pediatric patient.

_____ 10. Rubber dam isolation is not likely to be used in pediatric dentistry.

_____ 11. It is not necessary to use universal barrier techniques with a pediatric patient, since these patients do not fall into one of the high-risk categories.

_____ 12. Space maintainers are placed in the oral cavity to gain space lost by movement of teeth.

_____ 13. It is the responsibility of the dentist, not the dental assistant to observe signs of child abuse.

_____ 14. Nursing bottle mouth is seen only in children who are allowed to have a carbonated beverage in their bottles.

CRITICAL-THINKING ACTIVITIES

1. A child is seen in the pediatric office over a 6-month period, and the following details are evident during that time.
   a. Bruises on the child's head and neck area are evident on the front and the back sur-faces. The backs of his legs are often bruised.
   b. Bruise color ranges from bright blue to green to yellow.
   c. The child, even in warm weather, often wears long pants and long-sleeved shirts, there does not appear to be a cultural reason for this type of dress.
   d. The child is shy and withdrawn.

What is the significance of each of the preceding statements as it relates to possible child abuse. What questions might you ask the child, to determine his status?

2. You see a neighbor at a party. She knows you are a dental assistant and asks you about her 3-year-old daughter who has nursing bottle syndrome. The mother indicates that she has spoken to her dentist about the child's situation. The dentist has advised restoring all teeth and placing a space maintainer in an area where teeth have previously been extracted. The mother complains that it will cost too much money and that the child "will only lose the teeth in a couple of years anyway, so what is the point?"

What is your response to this mother? Be thorough in your explanation.

37 Periodontics

LEARNING OBJECTIVES

You will have mastered the material in this chapter when you can:

- Define the key terms
- Describe the role of the dental assistant in periodontics
- Describe types and signs of periodontal disease
- Record periodontal conditions, and state why each is important
- Identify and describe instruments and procedures used in periodontics
- Explain human relations practices that contribute to the success of periodontal treatment

KEY TERMS

Attachment width/AW
Bone swaging
Coronoplasty
Crevicular fluid
Curettage
Debridement
Digitized radiography
Donor tissue
Excise
False pocket
Festoon
Flap surgery
Furcation involvement
Gingivectomy
Gingivectomy knife
Gingivoplasty
Graft
Granulation tissue
Incise
Index
Infrabony pocket
Irrigation
Keyes technique
Mucogingival surgery
Mucoperiosteal flap
Mucosal flap
Occlusal equilibration
Osseous surgery
Oxygenating agent

Periodontal dressing
Periodontal surgery
Physiologic contour
Recession
Recipient tissue
Reflect
Resection
Root planing
Splint
Sulcular fluid
Sulcus temperature gauge
Suprabony pocket

FILL-IN QUESTIONS

Define the following terms

1. Subgingival curettage:

2. Sterile saline solution:

3. Flap procedure:

4. Pocket marker:

5. Identify three systemic and three dysfunctional factors that contribute to periodontal disease.

   Systemic

   a. _____

   b. _____

   c. _____

<u>Dysfunctional</u>

a. _____

b. _____

c. _____

6. List the appointment sequence for gingival surgery, and explain what is done at each appointment. Begin with consultation after diagnosis, and continue through initial recall after surgery.

7. Identify the instruments on the periodontal surgery tray pictured below.

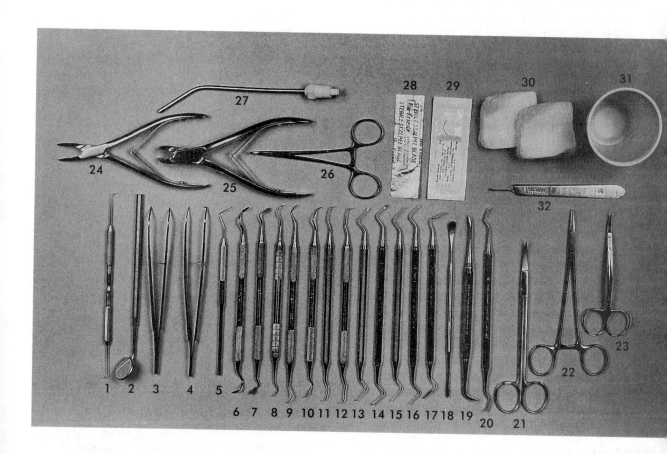

FIG. 37-1 Oral surgery tray setup.

MULTIPLE-CHOICE QUESTIONS

8. A modified sickle scaler is primarily used on the
   a. Interproximal surfaces of anterior teeth
   b. Interproximal surfaces of posterior teeth
   c. Interproximal surfaces of both anterior and posterior teeth
   d. Lingual and buccal surfaces

9. The following is true of the straight sickle scaler. It
   a. Is considered a universal scaler.
   b. Should not be used to remove subgingival calculus on the mandibular anterior teeth.
   c. Should not be used to remove supragingival calculus on the mandibular anterior teeth.
   d. Is used to remove posterior interproximal calculus.

10. The removal of calculus and portions of cementum to create a smooth hard root surface is referred to as
    a. Supragingival scaling
    b. Subgingival scaling
    c. Gross scaling
    d. Root planing

11. The major objective of scaling and root planing is to
    a. Create smooth root surfaces
    b. Create conditions that stimulate healthy gingival tissue
    c. Remove cementum
    d. Cause shrinkage of gingival tissue

12. The design shape of a curet scaler is similar to a(n)
    a. Ovoid
    b. Triangle
    c. Half-moon
    d. Rhomboid

13. Air may be used to deflect the free gingival margin, to detect
    a. Inflammation
    b. Subgingival calculus
    c. Supragingival calculus
    d. Smooth root surfaces

14. The primary function of a periodontal file is to
    a. Remove supragingival calculus
    b. Root plane
    c. Fracture heavy, tenacious calculus

15. An ultrasonic scaler should not remain on tooth structure very long, since it will
    a. Cause trauma to the gingival tissues
    b. Damage the tooth surface
    c. Cause the tip of the scaler to stop vibrating
    d. None of the above

16. After an ultrasonic scaler is used, it is necessary to use a manual scaler
    a. As a follow-up
    b. Only when directed by the dentist
    c. Only if scaling was difficult
    d. None of the above

17. A sharp dental instrument increases efficiency by
    1. Allowing the use of more lateral pressure
    2. Enhancing tactile sense
    3. Reducing trauma
    4. Decreasing the number of strokes that are necessary

    a. 1 and 3
    b. 2 and 4
    c. 2, 3, and 4
    d. 4 only

18. Which of the following procedures should be performed as part of the initial therapy phase of periodontal treatment?
    1. Oral hygiene instruction
    2. Temporary stabilization
    3. Removal of overhanging restorations
    4. Periodontal surgery
    5. Post-surgical evaluation

    a. 1, 2, and 4
    b. 1, 2, 3 and 5
    c. 2, 3, 4, and 5
    d. All of the above

19. Periodontal dressings are primarily used to
    1. Maintain the position of soft tissue
    2. Protect the soft tissues during flossing
    3. Promote healing
    4. Protect tooth structure from temperature changes
    5. Provide esthetics for the patient

    a. 1, 2, and 4
    b. 1, 3, and 4
    c. 2, 3, 4, and 5
    d. All of the above

20. Which of the following would be an acceptable diet for a patient after periodontal surgery?
    1. Normal diet, with care to eating habits
    2. Soft diet
    3. Crumbly diet for easier chewing
    4. Bland diet
    5. Nonirritative diet

    a. 1 and 2
    b. 1, 3, and 4
    c. 2, 4, and 5
    d. 1, 2, 4, and 5

21. The most important factor in the reduction of hypersensitivity is
    a. Minimized removal of tooth structure during root planing
    b. Use of home fluoride
    c. Professionally applied fluoride treatments
    d. Daily removal of all plaque from the mouth

CRITICAL-THINKING ACTIVITY

A patient who received periodontal treatment 1 week ago calls the office. She is concerned that her teeth are very sensitive, even more sensitive than they were before the surgery. The periodontist is unavailable to speak to the patient but has in the past directed you to address these patient concerns. What would you explain to the patient? Why are her teeth more sensitive, and what should she expect in the future? What can she do to help the in situation?

38   Forensic Dentistry

LEARNING OBJECTIVES

You will have mastered the material in this chapter when you can:

- Define the key terms
- Explain the importance of accurate patient records and radiographs to the identification of human remains
- Explain the process of dental identification of human remains
- Describe the role of the dental assistant in forensic odontology
- Explain the organization and duties of a forensic dental identification team
- Identify the armamentarium used in the identification of human remains
- Explain the rationale for marking of dental prostheses and appliances
- List situations when bite marks might occur
- List the protocol for bite mark case management
- List the components of child abuse and the likely subject of abuse
- List the signs of child abuse
- Explain the responsibilities for reporting suspected child abuse by health care professionals
- Explain the significance of forensic odontology to public service

KEY TERMS

Adjudication
Antemortem
Assailant
Coroner
Forensic anthropologist
Forensic odontology
Identification
Litigation
Mass disaster
Medical examiner
Perpetrator
Postmortem

FILL-IN QUESTIONS

1. List the four major areas in which forensic dentistry plays a major role.

   _____

   _____

   _____

   _____

2. Identify two areas in the dental office where the assistant assumes responsibility in forensic dentistry.

   _____

   _____

3. Identify the four sections of a forensic dental team, and explain the function of each section.

   Section:

   a. _____

   b. _____

   c. _____

   d. _____

   Function:

   a. _____

   b. _____

   c. _____

   d. _____

4. List the armamentarium that might be used in a forensic identification procedure:

5. List various behaviors that an abused child might display.

6. Describe the behavior of an abusive parent.

MULTIPLE-CHOICE QUESTIONS

7. Which of the following is *not* likely to be considered a reason to suspect child abuse?
   a. Lacerations of the lip, frenum, or uvula
   b. Torn labial frenum of child learning to walk
   c. Untreated fractures of teeth
   d. Oral burns

8. Which of the following could be considered suspect in potential child abuse situations?
   1. Markings of belts, belt buckles, cords or wires
   2. Bite and tooth marks on various areas of the body
   3. Bruises of assorted colors on dorsal aspect of legs and neck
   4. Bruises of a single color on the knees
   5. Lacerations on face and neck

   a. 1 and 3
   b. 2 and 4
   c. 1, 2, 3, and 4
   d. 1, 2, 3, and 5

TRUE OR FALSE QUESTIONS

Place a **T** for True or an **F** for False in the space provided as it refers to each statement.

_____ 9. Forensic dentistry is a recognized specialty of the ADA.

_____ 10. No two people, including identical twins, have the same dentition.

_____ 11. Every state requires that all newly fabricated removable prostheses contain identifying markings.

_____ 12. Health professionals in all states are mandated by law to report suspected abuse.

_____ 13. Reporting suspected abuse may prevent the additional suffering and possible death of an innocent person.

_____ 14. Failure to report child abuse may be considered a misdemeanor.

_____ 15. Tooth marks are recognized by the courts as providing proof of the assailant's identity.

CRITICAL-THINKING ACTIVITIES

1. Think back over the last 3 to 5 years, reflecting on the news of that period. In what local, state, or national disasters might a forensic dental team have been used to identify victims? Discuss the need for prompt identification in each of these situations, the impact of the incidents, and whether the news media referred to the need for a forensic dental team.

2. A patient who had been seen by a local dentist for many years for various types of restorative and preventive treatment is a victim in a tragic airline crash. To identify the body, the coroner requests premortem records. The records are presented, but no match of body remains can be confirmed because the documents from the dentist's office do not include routine radiographs or thorough clinical entries. What is the impact of this situation?

UNIT VIII

Laboratory Procedures

39   Basic Dental Laboratory Procedures

LEARNING OBJECTIVES

You will have mastered the material in this chapter when you can:

- Define the key terms
- Identify rules for safety in the laboratory
- Explain techniques for infection control in the laboratory
- Explain the use of a dental laboratory prescription or work order
- Describe the function of MSDS in relation to the laboratory
- Identify basic equipment used in the laboratory within a dental practice

KEY TERMS

Alcohol lamp
Articulator
Bunsen burner
Casting machine
Casting oven
Dental engine
Dental lathe
Gas torch
Gypsum bins
Investment oven
Laboratory prescription
Model trimmer
Sandblaster
Vacuum investing
Vacuum machine
Vibrator

FILL-IN QUESTIONS

1. List five common duties that a dental assistant might perform in the laboratory within the dental office.

   _____

   _____

   _____

   _____

   _____

2. List eight safety rules that should be practiced when working in the laboratory.

   _____

   _____

   _____

   _____

   _____

   _____

   _____

3. Describe the steps that should be taken to prevent the transmission of disease from the laboratory to the office.

   _____

   _____

   _____

   _____

   _____

   _____

   _____

4. What information does OSHA require to appear on MSDS forms?

_____

_____

_____

_____

_____

_____

_____

_____

_____

5. Select five materials that are found in your clinic or office and enter the appropriate data for each of these products in the spaces below.

Substance #1

Chemical _____

Product _____

Manufacturer _____

Generic area _____

MSDS on file _____

Substance #2

Chemical _____

Product _____

Manufactuer _____

Generic area _____

MSDS on file _____

Substance #3

Chemical _____

Product _____

Manufacturer _____

Generic area _____

MSDS on file _____

Substance #3

Chemical _____

Product _____

Manufacturer _____

Generic area _____

MSDS on file _____

Substance #4

Chemical _____

Product _____

Manufacturer _____

Generic area _____

MSDS on file _____

Substance #5

Chemical _____

Product _____

Manufacturer _____

Generic area _____

MSDS on file _____

MATCHING QUESTIONS

Choose the term that best identifies each of the following the descriptions.

a. Alcohol lamp   e. Articulator
b. Bunsen burner   f. Casting machine
c. Casting oven   g. Dental engine
d. Dental lathe   h. Gas torch

_____ 6. May be used with a rag wheel to polish a denture

_____ 7. Portable flame

_____ 8. Available in quadrant, full-arch, or condylar styles

_____ 9. Heats a ring from which a metal crown can be made

_____ 10. Provides a source of heat to melt metal for a casting

_____ 11. A source of energy for a handpiece and various rotary instruments

TRUE OR FALSE QUESTIONS

Place a **T** or an **F** in the space provided as it refers to the following statements.

_____ 12. All manufacturers of products that contain hazardous chemicals are legally obligated to provide the MSDS sheets for each product at the time of shipping to the purchaser.

_____ 13. The OSHA Hazard Communication Standard, Title 29, Code of Federal Regulations 1910.1200, requires that all dental professionals take certain steps to comply with the standard.

_____ 14. MSDS is the acronym for Material Safety Data Standards.

_____ 15. Nippers may be used to contour the cervical margins of a metal casting.

_____ 16. The consumption of food or smoking in areas where chemicals are used is not allowed.

_____ 17. All hazardous chemicals must be disposed of in accordance with MSDS instructions and applicable federal regulations.

_____ 18. Certain products that are regulated by the Food and Drug Administration (FDA), such as impression materials, are exempt from the Hazard Communication Standard.

_____ 19. When chemicals are transferred from the original container to a smaller container for use in the dental office, only the name of the product and generic origin need be transferred to the new container.

_____ 20. Employers are required to provide employees with a one-time-only information and training seminar on all hazardous chemicals found in the dental office.

CLINICAL APPLICATION

1. Complete the laboratory requisition form below, using the information obtained from the following patient clinical record. The patient is Mrs. Rebecca Fitzgerald, age 49 years. She is to have a fixed bridge constructed, replacing the mandibular right first molar. The mesial abutment is a three-quarter crown, and the distal abutment a full crown. The distal abutment and the pontic are to be of porcelain fused to metal. The record indicates the shade is Bioform 65 and that the castings are to be made of nonprecious metal. The doctor prefers to "try in" the abutment crowns before soldering. The try-in should be performed at 2 weeks from this date. A final seating 1 week later is preferred. Provide the necessary data to complete the form. Information about the dentist includes the following: Joseph W. Lake, 255 North Tucker St., Duluth, Ohio 43476, license number 0030OH

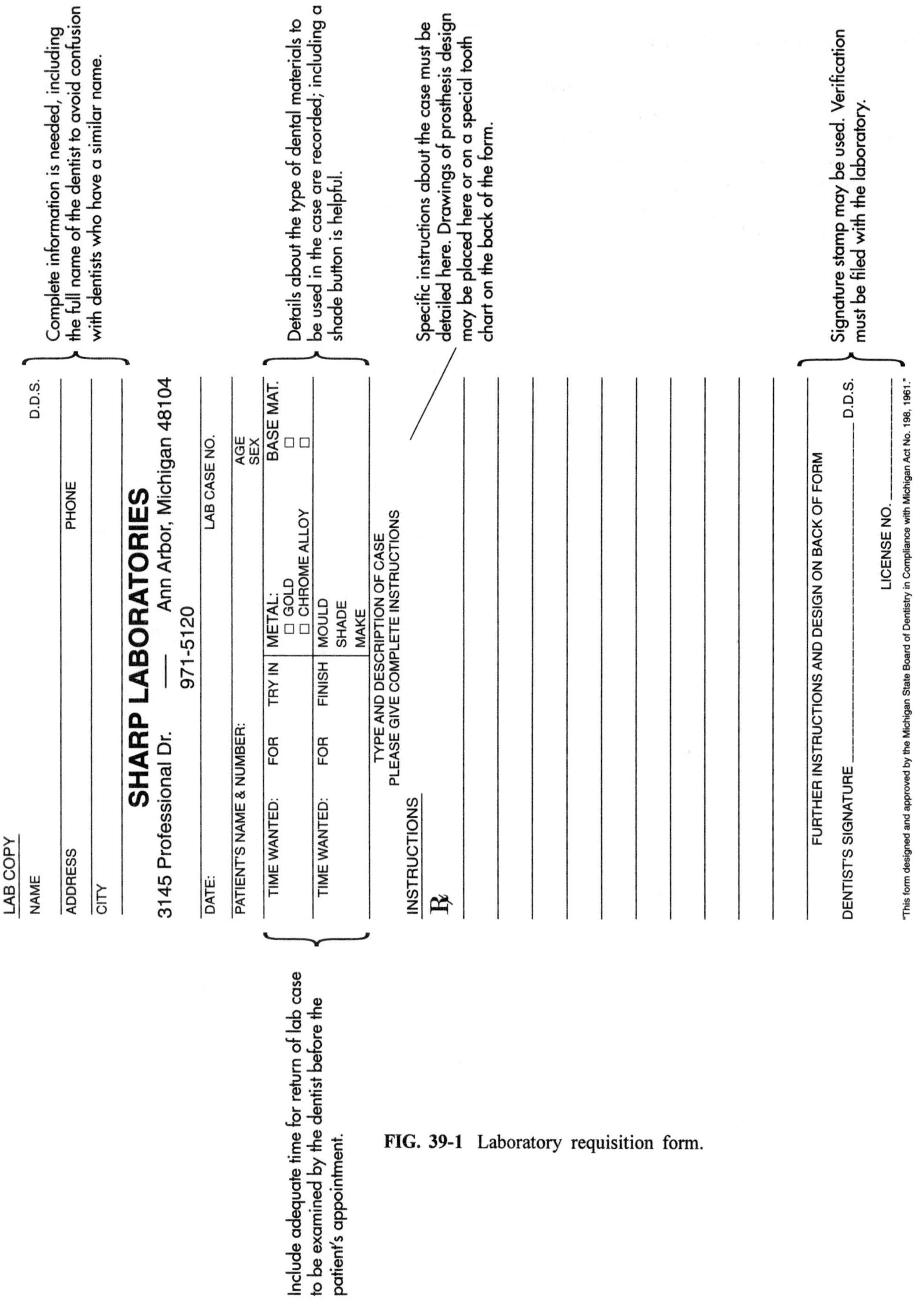

Complete information is needed, including the full name of the dentist to avoid confusion with dentists who have a similar name.

Details about the type of dental materials to be used in the case are recorded; including a shade button is helpful.

Specific instructions about the case must be detailed here. Drawings of prosthesis design may be placed here or on a special tooth chart on the back of the form.

Signature stamp may be used. Verification must be filed with the laboratory.

LAB COPY

NAME _____ D.D.S.

ADDRESS _____ PHONE

CITY

SHARP LABORATORIES

3145 Professional Dr. ——— Ann Arbor, Michigan 48104

971-5120

DATE: _____ LAB CASE NO.

PATIENT'S NAME & NUMBER: _____ AGE _____ SEX _____

| TIME WANTED: | FOR | TRY IN | METAL: ☐ GOLD ☐ CHROME ALLOY | BASE MAT. ☐ ☐ |
| TIME WANTED: | FOR | FINISH | MOULD SHADE MAKE | |

TYPE AND DESCRIPTION OF CASE
PLEASE GIVE COMPLETE INSTRUCTIONS

INSTRUCTIONS

℞ _____

_____

_____

_____

_____

_____

_____

_____

_____

_____

FURTHER INSTRUCTIONS AND DESIGN ON BACK OF FORM

DENTIST'S SIGNATURE _____ D.D.S.

LICENSE NO. _____

"This form designed and approved by the Michigan State Board of Dentistry in Compliance with Michigan Act No. 198, 1961."

Include adequate time for return of lab case to be examined by the dentist before the patient's appointment.

FIG. 39-1 Laboratory requisition form.

184

CRITICAL-THINKING ACTIVITY

In preparing to transfer the previously described patient to the laboratory a final impression, an opposing impression, a bite registration, and the shade button must be sent. What steps would you follow in preparation to transfer this patient? What risks are there in transferring a patient from the dental office to the laboratory?

40   Advanced Dental Laboratory Procedures

LEARNING OBJECTIVES

You will have mastered the material in this chapter when you can:

- Define the key terms
- Define the purpose of diagnostic models
- Explain the procedure for pouring an alginate impression with a gypsum product for the purpose of creating a diagnostic model
- Identify the criteria for poured models
- Describe and demonstrate the procedure for trimming diagnostic models
- Explain the criteria for trimmed diagnostic models
- Explain the advantages for using a custom made tray
- Describe and demonstrate the procedure for construction of custom-made trays
- Explain the criteria for clinically acceptable custom-made trays
- Explain the function of a mouthguard
- Describe the construction of a mouthguard
- Explain the criteria for a clinically acceptable mouthguard
- Describe the process of repairing a denture
- Describe the construction of a baseplate

KEY TERMS

Anatomic portion
Angle former
Art portion
Base
Custom-made tray
Diagnostic model
Mouthguard
Parallel
Spacer
Symmetric

FILL-IN QUESTIONS

1. The portion of a diagnostic model that includes the teeth and supporting structures is referred to as the _____ portion, and the base of the model is the _____ portion.

2. The imaginary concave line that is formed on the mandibular dentition along the occlusal surface from the canine to the third molar is referred to as the _____.

3. List six purposes for the use of diagnostic models.

   _____

   _____

   _____

   _____

   _____

   _____

4. Impressions are a _____ reproduction of the intraoral anatomy, and the final result—the set of diagnostic models—is a _____ reproduction.

5. List five criteria for properly poured models.

   _____

   _____

   _____

   _____

6. List 10 criteria for properly trimmed models.

   _____

   _____

   _____

   _____

_____

_____

_____

_____

_____

7. Identify three factors that can alter the method of trimming a set of models.

_____

_____

_____

8. Identify five advantages of using a custom-made tray rather than a stock tray during a final impression.

_____

_____

_____

_____

_____

9. List 10 characteristics of a clinically acceptable custom-made acrylic tray.

_____

_____

_____

_____

_____

_____

_____

_____

10. Identify five characteristics of a clinically acceptable mouthguard.

_____

_____

_____

_____

_____

MATCHING QUESTIONS

Select the term that best defines the cut or angle described in each of the following statements.

   a. Symmetric
   b. Parallel
   c. Curved

_____ 11. Anterior of mandibular model
_____ 12. Backs of articulated models
_____ 13. Angle of the heels of maxillary model
_____ 14. Angle of the sides of both models
_____ 15. Anterior cuts of maxillary model

MULTIPLE-CHOICE QUESTIONS

16. Diagnostic models are generally poured in which of the following materials?
   a. Plaster
   b. Class I stone
   c. Class II stone
   d. Investment

17. When model trimming is begun, the first arch to be trimmed is the following:
   a. Maxillary
   b. Mandibular

18. The placement of stops on custom-made trays is necessary
   a. For the release of impression materials
   b. For definitive placement of the tray in the mouth
   c. Only on the anterior portion of the tray
   d. Only on the posterior portion of the tray

19. A custom-made tray for an edentulous model should extend
    a. 2 mm short of the peripheral roll
    b. 2 mm beyond the peripheral roll
    c. 2 mm below the frenum
    d. To the deepest portion of the peripheral roll

20. Before trimming, models should be soaked for
    a. 1 to 2 minutes
    b. 5 minutes
    c. 10 minutes
    d. 20 minutes

21. Which of the following statements include information that is necessary for labeling diagnostic models.
    1. Type labels for both models.
    2. Include the patient's name and age at the time of the impression
    3. Include the date of the impression
    4. Include the date of trimming

    a. 1 and 3
    b. 2 and 4
    c. 1, 2, and 3
    d. All of the above

22. The use of a mouthguard during contact sports can do all *except*
    a. Prevent tooth injury by absorbing and deflecting blows to the teeth.
    b. Prevent jaw fractures by creating a cushion between the teeth during the impact of the blow.
    c. Protect oral tissues from laceration by shielding the lips, tongue, and gingival tissues.
    d. Reduce potential TMJ disorders by cushioning the upper jaw.
    e. Prevent potential concussions by absorbing the shock of a blow to the mandible.

TRUE OR FALSE QUESTIONS

In the space provided place a **T** for True or an **F** for False as it relates to each statement.

_____ 23. The bases of a trimmed set of diagnostic models should be parallel to each other.
_____ 24. During trimming the table of the model trimmer should be at a 45-degree angle to the cutting wheel of the model trimmer.

_____ 25. A self-curing acrylic is used to construct a custom-made tray.
_____ 26. When a full-arch mandibular tray is being constructed, the softened acrylic material is first adapted to the tongue space.
_____ 27. Acrylic material that is used to create a custom-made tray should be of uniform thickness.

CLINICAL APPLICATION

1. The model is divided into two parts, the anatomic and the art portions. In general the anatomic portion equals two thirds of the total height of the model, and the art portion, one third. If the depth of the mucolabial fold at the cuspid region on the right side is 27 and on the left side is 29, what will be the measurements for each of the following?

   Anatomic portion _____
   Art portion _____
   Total height of maxillary model _____
   Total height of articulated models _____

2. A patient is seen in the dental office after breaking a mandibular denture into two parts. The break is at the midline of the anterior. Explain the steps necessary to repair this denture.

CRITICAL-THINKING ACTIVITY

Indicate which lines must be cut to make the model symmetric in the following drawing.

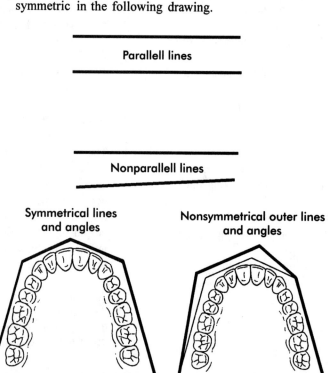

Parallell lines

Nonparallell lines

Symmetrical lines and angles

Nonsymmetrical outer lines and angles

FIG. 40-1 Lines and angles illustrate parallelism and symmetry.

EPILOGUE

41   The Beginning: Marketing Your Skills

LEARNING OBJECTIVES

You will have mastered the material in this chapter when you can:

- Determine your career goals
- Identify your personal assets and liabilities for a job
- Determine desirable characteristics for a job you might seek
- Identify personal priorities for a potential job
- Determine methods of marketing your skills
- Prepare data for job applications and interviews
- Explain how to advance on the job

CRITICAL THINKING

1. Spend some time thinking about the type of job you want. Ask yourself questions such as the following:
   a. In what type of environment am I happiest? Environments include the following: a large clinic; a small family-type practice; specialty or general practice; working with adults, children, persons with special needs, or older adults; and a small-volume or large-volume practice.
   b. What type of people challenge me the most? With whom am I the most comfortable? Think back over your life, and identify the people who have had the greatest impact on you. What was so special about these people? Consider that they might represent the type of people with whom you want to work.
   c. What part of dental assisting excites me the most—Chairside, business office, laboratory, or the variety? Will I be satisfied doing just one task?
   d. Where do I want to be in my career a year from now? Five years from now?

2. Spend some time by yourself and then with a peer or teacher who knows you well. Identify several strengths and weaknesses that you have for a potential job. How can you overcome your weaknesses? Are you willing to exert the effort to improve?

3. Prepare data to be used in completing a job application. You might consider preparing a small notebook that could be taken with you to an interview. Include complete personal data; names, addresses, and phone numbers of references; previous job information; a list of job priorities, and questions you wish to ask during the interview.

4. Imagine that you are a recent graduate of a dental assistant program, have a credential from DANB, and have been offered a job with the basic duties you are seeking. The dentist suggests that your starting salary will be $8.50 per hour and that health care and HBV immunization are the benefits for the first year. At the end of 1 year a merit evaluation will be completed, but whether there is potential for advancement and whether other benefits will be offered later are uncertain. What is your reaction to this offer? How does this salary compare to that of local allied health care workers with similar education and experience? How does it compare with studies done by the ADA? How does it compare with various economic levels in your area and in the United States? Consider how you might respond to this offer in a professional manner, and explain how you would do so.

CHAPTER ANSWERS

CHAPTER 1

1. American Dental Association
2. Certified Dental Assistant
3. Certified Dental Technician
4. Certified Orthodontic Assistant
5. Certified Dental Practice Management Assistant
6. Certified Oral and Maxillofacial Surgery Assistant
7. Doctor of Dental Surgery
8. Dental Assistant National Board
9. Registered Dental Assistant
10. Registered Dental Assistant in Expanded Functions
11. Registered Dental Hygienist
12. Doctor of Dental Medicine
13. a. Endodontics
    b. Oral Maxillofacial surgery
    c. Oral pathology
    d. Orthodontics
    e. Pediatric dentistry
    f. Periodontics
    g. Prosthetics
    h. Public health dentistry
14. a. Public health dentist
    b. Orthodontist
    c. Endodontist
    d. Periodontist
    e. Pediatric dentist
15. a. Dentist
    b. Dental assistant
    c. Dental hygienist
    d. Dental laboratory technician
16. The patient
17. -ics
18. -ist
19. Refer to chapter 1 of text for detailed descriptions.
20. b
21. d
22. a
23. f
24. b
25. d
26. d

CHAPTER 2

1. Refer to Chapter 2 for detailed descriptions.
2. Edmund Kells
3. Minnesota
4. a
5. a

CHAPTER 3

1. Aids in mastication
   Aids in facial expression
2. Ptyalin
3. a. Maxillary sinus
   b. Close to maxillary molars roots during oral surgery and related pain associated with sinusitis
4. Any two of the following:
   Lighten the skull
   Provide resonance to the voice
   Warm the respirated air
5. Lingual branch of the external carotid artery
6. Trigeminal nerve
7. Mandibular division
8. Frontal, occipital, sphenoid, temporal, ethmoid, parietal
9. Mandible, vomer, nasal bones, zygomatic bones, inferior nasal conchae, palatine bones, maxillae
10. Name the structures indicated by each line (frontal view of the skull).
11. Name the structures indicated by each line (lateral view of the skull).
12. Name the structures indicated by each line (inferior view of the skull).
13. Name the structures indicated by each line (TMJ diagram).
14. Name the structures indicated by each line (lateral view of the muscle structure).
15. Name the structures indicated by each line (frontal view of the sinuses).
16. Name the structures indicated by each line (lateral view of the sinuses).
17. Name the structures indicated by each line (frontal view of the face).
18. Name the structures indicated by each line (open mouth).
19. a
20. c
21. e
22. b
23. g
24. c
25. d
26. h
27. f
28. i
29. b
30. f
31. a
32. b
33. b
34. b

35. F
36. F
37. T
38. T
39. T
40. T
41. F

CHAPTER 4

1. 32
2. 20
3. Central incisor, lateral incisor, canine, first premolar, second premolar, first molar, second molar, third molar

UNIVERSAL (ADA)	PALMER	FDI
4. 32	8⌐	48
5. 30	6⌐	46
6. 24	⌐1	31
7. 28	4⌐	44
8. T	T̄⌐	85
9. 8	A⌐	21
10. Q	B⌐	82

11. #19, #3
12. a. Ameloblast
    b. Fibroblast
    c. Cementoblast
    d. Odontoblast
13. Refer to Chapter 4 for complete descriptions.
14. a. 10 years of age
    b. 8-33 months of age
    c. 7 years of age
    d. 15+ years of age
15. Name the structures indicated by each line (diagram of tooth).
16. Name the structures indicated by each line. Be specific (diagram of the permanent dentition).
17. b
18. c
19. e
20. c
21. d
22. a
23. b
24. b
25. e
26. c
27. a
28. e
29. d
30. f

31. b
32. a
33. b
34. b
35. b
36. c
37. a
38. c
39. b
40. a
41. d
42. b

CHAPTER 5

1. Refer to Chapter 5 for a complete description.
2. Refer to Chapter 5 for a complete description.
3. a. Major
   b. Major
   c. Major
   d. Major
   e. Major
   f. Major
   g. Trace
   h. Trace
   i. Trace
   j. Major
   k. Trace
   l. Trace
4. Refer to Chapter 5 for a complete description.
5. Refer to Chapter 5 for a complete description.
6. Refer to Chapter 5 for a complete description.
7. Diet beverage, substitute for sweet relish
8. c
9. d
10. d
11. a
12. c
13. b
14. a
15. a

CHAPTER 6

1. Refer to Chapter 6 for a complete description.
2. Refer to Chapter 6 for a complete description.
3. b
4. a
5. e
6. b
7. a
8. c
9. c
10. c

11. c
12. d
13. b
14. F
15. T
16. F
17. T
18. T
19. F
20. T
21. T

CHAPTER 7

1. Heat, redness, pain, swelling
2. Refer to Chapter 7 for complete description.
3. Excessive growth of tissue.
4. 1) Compare opposite sides for similarities or differences.
   2) If opposites are the same the condition may be normal for that patient.
   3) Obtain a history of the lesion.
5. Refer to Chapter 7 for complete description.
6. Refer to Chapter 7 for complete description.
7. Xerostomia and radiation caries
8. Refer to Chapter 7 for complete description.
9. e
10. f
11. a
12. i
13. m
14. h
15. c
16. d
17. g
18. b
19. k
20. b
21. c
22. d
23. d
24. c
25. b
26. d
27. c
28. c
29. d
30. b
31. c
32. a
33. b
34. c
35. b
36. a

CHAPTER 8

1. Refer to chapter 08 for a complete description.
2. Refer to chapter 08 for a complete description.
3. Refer to chapter 08 for a complete description.
4. Refer to chapter 08 for a complete description.
5. Refer to chapter 08 for a complete description.
6. Steam under pressure
   Time: 15 to 20 min
   Temperature: 240° to 260°
   Pressure: 15 to 20 lb
   Dry heat
   Time: 1 hour
   Temperature 320° to 350°
   Pressure: 0 lb
   Chemical vapor
   Time: 20 min
   Temperature: Preset
   Pressure 20 lb
7. Occupational Safety and Health Administration/Act
8. Dental health care worker
9. Acquired immunodeficiency syndrome
10. Centers for Disease Control and Prevention
11. Environmental protection agency
12. Hepatitis B virus
13. Human immunodeficiency virus
14. Refer to Chapter 8 for complete description.
15. Refer to Chapter 8 for complete description.
16. Refer to Chapter 8 for complete description.
17. Refer to Chapter 8 for complete description.
18. a. 3
    b. 1
    c. 2
19. Refer to Chapter 8 for complete description.
20. Refer to Chapter 8 for complete description.
21. Refer to Chapter 8 for complete description.
22. b
23. c
24. d
25. e
26. a
27. b
28. a
29. e
30. b
31. b
32. b
33. b
34. e
35. c
36. a
37. h
38. d

39. g
40. e
41. e
42. b
43. b
44. b
45. c
46. e
47. d
48. b
49. b
50. d
51. b
52. e
53. b
54. b
55. a
56. F
57. F
58. F
59. F
60. F
61. F
62. T
63. F
64. F
65. F

CHAPTER 9

1. Refer to Chapter 9 for a complete description.
2. Refer to Chapter 9 for a complete description.
3. Refer to Chapter 9 for a complete description.
4. Refer to Chapter 9 for a complete description.
5. Refer to Chapter 9 for a complete description.
6. Refer to Chapter 9 for a complete description.
7. Refer to Chapter 9 for a complete description.
8. Refer to Chapter 9 for a complete description.
9. Cone cut. Position the PID so that the central ray is centered in the middle of the film.
10. Elongation. Change the vertical angulation of the PID.
11. Foreshortening. Change the vertical angulation of the PID>.
12. Dark film. Film is overexposed or overdeveloped.
13. Fogged film. Light exposure occurred during processing.
14. Herringbone effect. Film is placed with the lead sheet closest to the image instead of away from the image.
15. Overlapping (bite-wing). Change horizontal angulation.

16. Crescent mark. Film was bent before or during exposure.
17. Film brand, speed, size of film, side closest to the PID, mounting dot
18. Refer to Chapter 8 for a complete description.
19. Refer to Chapter 8 for a complete description.
20. b
21. b
22. a
23. b
24. a
25. b
26. b
27. c
28. b
29. d
30. b
31. b
32. a
33. a
34. c
35. a
36. b
37. b
38. a
39. b
40. c

CHAPTER 10

1. Dyspnea
2. Rapid, slow
3. PDR, USP, NF
4. Analgesic, antibiotic, tranquilizer, vasoconstrictor
5. The name of the drug other than the trade name
6. The name a manufacturer gives to the drug
7. g
8. m
9. h
10. j
11. k
12. e
13. c
14. l
15. b
16. d
17. f
18. m
19. l
20. k
21. d
22. e
23. a

24. j
25. b
26. d
27. c
28. d
29. d
30. c
31. d
32. b

CHAPTER 11

1. e
2. r
3. r
4. e
5. r
6. e
7. e
8. e
9. e
10. e
11. Agar hydrocolloid
12. Refer to Chapter 11 for a complete description.
13. Refer to Chapter 11 for a complete description.
14. Monomers, polymers, polymerization
15. Mercury
16. Refer to Chapter 11 for a complete description.
17. Refer to Chapter 11 for a complete description.
18. Refer to Chapter 11 for a complete description.
19. Refer to Chapter 11 for a complete description.
20. e
21. d
22. l
23. b
24. g
25. l
26. k
27. e
28. j
29. a
30. i
31. h
32. c
33. a
34. c
35. d
36. a
37. a
38. b
39. b
40. c
41. c
42. a

43. b
44. a
45. c
46. c
47. b
48. b
49. b
50. b
51. c
52. a
53. a
54. c
55. a
56. d
57. a
58. c
59. c
60. a
61. d
62. b
63. a
64. a
65. b
66. b
67. c
68. T
69. T
70. F
71. F
72. F
73. T
74. F
75. F
76. T
77. T
78. T
79. F
80. F

CHAPTER 12

1. Implied and informed
2. Refer to Chapter 12 for a complete descriptions.
3. Refer to Chapter 12 for a complete descriptions.
4. Refer to Chapter 12 for a complete descriptions.
5. Refer to Chapter 12 for a complete descriptions.
6. Refer to Chapter 12 for a complete descriptions.
7. b
8. b
9. c
10. b
11. a
12. e
13. d

14. e
15. c
16. g
17. b
18. a
19. e
20. f
21. h
22. k
23. i
24. g
25. j
26. l
27. m
28. n
29. d
30. r
31. s
32. p
33. o
34. q
35. a
36. a
37. c
38. T
39. T
40. T
41. F
42. T
43. T
44. T

CHAPTER 13

1. Levels of Maslow's hierarchy
   Physiologic, biologic
   Safety, security
   Social, love
   Esteem
   Self-actualization
2. Communication
3. Any of the following:
   Self-confidence
   Genuineness
   Openness to experience
   Acceptance of backgrounds and values of others
   Enthusiasm
   Integrity
   Assertiveness
   Effective listening
   Sense of humor
   Recognition of the needs of others
4. Any of the list below:
   Criticizing

Name calling
Diagnosing
Praising evaluatively
Ordering
Threatening
Questioning
Advising
Diverting
Ignoring
5. Refer to Chapter 13 for a complete description.
6. Refer to Chapter 13 for a complete description.
7. b
8. c
9. b
10. d
11. a

CHAPTER 14

1. Pegboard and computer
2. Refer to Chapter 14 for a complete description.
3. Protection of both the patient and dentist
   Information for tax purposes
   Data for business analysis
4. a. Contains listing of activities for each patient seen during the day
   b. Contains financial information for each patient or family
   c. Request for payment
   d. Provides storage for ledger cards
   e. Multiple-copy receipt/charge form that can serve as a copy for the patient, insurance carrier and office
5. Refer to Chapter 14 for a complete description.
6. Mail, telephone, and advanced appointment
7. Refer to Chapter 14 for a complete description.
8. Refer to Chapter 14 for a complete description.
9. Padding fees
   Billing before completion of treatment
   Predating or postdating claim forms
   Falsely listing treatment that was rendered
   Not working within the contract
10. c
11. a
12. a
13. d
14. c
15. e
16. e
17. b
18. c
19. c
20. b
21. c

22. d
23. c
24. F
25. T
26. T
27. F
28. T
29. T
30. c
31. a
32. b
33. d
34. a
35. f
36. e
37. b
38. c
39. d
40. i

CHAPTER 15

1. Finger only; fingers, wrist, and elbow; movement of torso
2. Refer to Chapter 15 for a complete description.
3. Refer to Chapter 15 for a complete description.
4. d
5. c
6. T
7. F
8. T
9. T
10. F
11. T
12. T
13. T

CHAPTER 16

1. Refer to Chapter 16 for a complete description.
2. Refer to Chapter 16 for a complete description.
3. m
4. g
5. l
6. b
7. n
8. i
9. a
10. h
11. f
12. c
13. k
14. c
15. f

16. e
17. g
18. d
19. b
20. a
21. c
22. d

CHAPTER 17

1. Refer to Chapter 17 for a complete description.
2. Refer to Chapter 17 for a complete description.
3. Refer to Chapter 17 for a complete description.
4. Refer to Chapter 17 for a complete description.
5. d
6. d
7. T
8. T
9. F
10. F
11. F
12. T
13. T
14. F
15. T

CHAPTER 18

1. Straight, monangle, binagle, triple angle
2. Illumination, retraction, indirect vision
3. e
4. a
5. d
6. n
7. m
8. l
9. j
10. g
11. i
12. c
13. b
14. h
15. a
16. b
17. b
18. c
19. a
20. T
21. T
22. F
23. F

CHAPTER 19

1. a. 33½ to 43
    b. ¼ to 10
    c. 55 to 64
    d. 555 to 564
    e. 169 to 172 (69 to 72)
    f. 700 to 708
2. a. Round
    b. Small round
    c. Round or inverted cone
    d. Straight or tapered fissure plain cut
    e. Tapered fissure cross cut or special depth groove bur
3. a. Round
    b. Tapered fissure plain cut
    c. Inverted cone
    d. Straight fissure cross cut
    e. Tapered fissure cross cut
    f. Wheel
    g. Straight fissure plain cut
4. Cutting surface is toward the shank.
5. Cutting surface is away from the shank.
6. j
7. n
8. i
9. c
10. a
11. b
12. g
13. m
14. d
15. f
16. e
17. c
18. c
19. c
20. c
21. F
22. F
23. F
24. T
25. T
26. T
27. T
28. T
29. F
30. F

CHAPTER 20

1. Pen grasp, modified pen grasp, palm grasp

2. Transfer portion: thumb, forefinger, and middle finger
    Receiving portion: fourth and five fingers
3. Left, right, right, left
4. Refer to Chapter 20 for a complete description.
5. a, d, b, e, f, c, g, j, h, k, i
6. c
7. a
8. b (optional a)
9. a
10. a
11. a
12. a
13. a
14. b (optional a)
15. e
16. d
17. T
18. F
19. T
20. F
21. F
22. T
23. F
24. F
25. T
26. F

CHAPTER 21

1. Refer to Chapter 21 for a complete description.
2. Refer to Chapter 21 for a complete description.
3. Refer to Chapter 21 for a complete description.
4. Refer to Chapter 21 for a complete description.
5. Refer to Chapter 21 for a complete description.
6. c
7. d
8. c
9. a
10. c
11. d
12. a
13. d
14. d
15. d
16. a
17. b

CHAPTER 22

1. Refer to Chapter 22 for a complete description.
2. Refer to Chapter 22 for a complete description.
3. Refer to Chapter 22 for a complete description.
4. Refer to Chapter 22 for a complete description.

5. c
6. b
7. a
8. b
9. a
10. e
11. b
12. b
13. i
14. d
15. k
16. e
17. l
18. g
19. n
20. m
21. b

CHAPTER 23

1. a. Short, 30 ga
   b. Short, 30 ga
   c. Long, 27 ga
   c. Long, 27 ga
2. a. Hub
   b. Harpoon
   c. Plunger
   d. Barrel
   e. Finger rest
   f. Thumb ring
3. a. Infiltration
   b. Field block
   c. Field block (Some circumstances nerve block)
   d. Nerve block
4. Refer to Chapter 23 for a complete description.
5. c
6. g
7. l
8. a
9. b
10. j
11. d
12. m
13. e
14. f
15. k
16. c
17. c
18. c
19. b
20. a
21. a. 2
    b. 5

c. 3
d. 9
e. 6
f. 8
g. 7
h. 4
i. 1

CHAPTER 24

1. Refer to Chapter 24 for complete descriptions.
2. Refer to Chapter 24 for complete descriptions.
3. Refer to Chapter 24 for complete descriptions.
4. Refer to Chapter 24 for complete descriptions.
5. Refer to Chapter 24 for complete descriptions.
6. Refer to Chapter 24 for complete descriptions.
7. Refer to Chapter 24 for complete descriptions.
8. Refer to Chapter 24 for complete descriptions.
9. Refer to Chapter 24 for complete descriptions.
10. Refer to Chapter 24 for complete descriptions.
11. f
12. g
13. d
14. a
15. d
16. d
17. b
18. b
19. d
20. c
21. d
22. d
23. a
24. b
25. c
26. T
27. T
28. F
29. F
30. T
31. F
32. F
33. T

CHAPTER 25

1. Refer to Chapter 25 for a complete description.
2. Refer to Chapter 25 for a complete description.
3. b
4. e
5. g
6. d
7. h
8. a

9. c
10. a
11. a
12. c
13. c
14. b
15. b
16. c
17. b
18. b
19. b

CHAPTER 26

1. Refer to Chapter 26 for a complete description.
2. Refer to Chapter 26 for a complete description.
3. Prevention of oral disease
4. Plaque, stain and calculus
5. Refer to Chapter 26 for a complete description.
6. Refer to Chapter 26 for a complete description.
7. k
8. l
9. e
10. m
11. g
12. d
13. j
14. b
15. i
16. c
17. a
18. d
19. c
20. f
21. b
22. g
23. a
24. b
25. b
26. b
27. c
28. c
29. b
30. b

CHAPTER 27

1. a. Explorer
   b. Smooth surface carver such as Ward's or Hollenback explorer
   c. Large cleoid-discoid (7C), or 26 spoon
   d. FG bur such as No. 34 or No. 2
   e. Small cleoid-discoid (5C), burnisher, explorer

f. Enamel hatchet
g. Cavity varnish
h. Small FG round bur
i. Burnisher (ball or other)
j. Mirror handle
k. Amalgam carrier/gun syringe
l. Large condensor
m. Plastic instrument, No. 25 Wesco condensor
n. Wedge
o. Gingival marginal trimmer
p. Articulating paper
q. Fissure bur
r. Spoon excavator
s. Low speed handpiece with round bur
t. Matrix band and retainer
u. Amalgamator

2. a. No. 34 or No. 2 FG, high speed
   b. No. 55 to 64 FG, high speed
   c. No. ¼ to 1 FG/RA, high or low speed
   d. Usually No. 2 to No. 8 FG/RA, low speed
3. Adapt the matrix band to the tooth.
   Create larger interproximal space.
4. Occlusal aspect;
   a. vise
   b. frame
   c. inner knob
   d. outer knob
   Gingival aspect
   e. guide slots
   f. diagonal slot
5. 1. Explorer
   2. Mirror
   3. Cotton pliers
   4. Spoon excavator
   5. Enamel hatchet
   6. Mesial gingival marginal trimmer
   7. Distal gingival marginal trimmer
   8. Amalgam carrier
   9. No. 1 condenser
   10. No. 2 condenser
   11. No. 7 Cleoid-discoid carver
   12. Ward's carver
   13. No. 5 Cleoid-discoid carver
   14. No. 21 B anatomic burnisher
   15. Ball burnisher
   16. Articulating paper holder
   17. Thumb forceps
   18. HVE tip
   19. Beavertail burnisher
   20. Hollenback carver
   21. Smooth and anatomic carver
   22. Back-action condenser
   23. Wesco 25

24. Articulating paper
25. 2-by-2" gauze
26. Patient napkin chain
27. Wedges
28. Plastic film divider to mix liners
29. Tofflemire matrix band and retainer
30. A/W syringe tip
31. A/W syringe tip cover
32. Cotton pellets
33. Dappen dish
34. Assorted burs
35. Cotton rolls

6. Refer to Chapter 27 for a complete description.
7. c
8. h
9. l
10. f
11. j
12. i
13. d
14. e
15. b
16. a
17. b
18. e
19. F
20. F
21. F
22. T
23. T
24. F
25. F
26. F
27. F
28. T
29. F
30. T
31. F
32. T
33. T

CHAPTER 28

1. Refer to Chapter 28 for a complete description.
2. Refer to Chapter 28 for a complete description.
3. 1. Explorer
   2. Mirror
   3. Cotton pliers
   4. Spoon excavator
   5. Binangle chisel
   6. Wedelstaedt chisel
   7. Plastic teflon instrument
   8. Linen strip
   9. HVE tip

10. No. 12B scalpel blade and handle
11. Thumb forceps
12. Bur block with burs and stones
13. Mylar/celluloid strip
14. Bur tool
15. Dappen dish
16. Articulating paper
17. A/W tip
18. A/W tip cover
19. Cotton pellets
20. Cotton rolls
21. Floss
22. Wedge
23. Matrix strip holder
24. Napkin chain
25. 2-by-2" gauze

4. d
5. c
6. a
7. c
8. a
9. a
10. d
11. c
12. c
13. a
14. T
15. T
16. T
17. F

CHAPTER 29

1. Refer to Chapter 29 for a complete description.
2. a. Inlay
   b. Onlay
   c. 3/4 crown
   d. Full crown
   e. Fixed bridge
   f. Dental laminate
   g. Full porcelain
   h. Cantilever bridge
   i. Maryland bridge
3. a. Drifting of adjacent teeth
   b. Hypereruption of opposing teeth
   c. Food impaction
   d. Dental caries
   e. Periodontal disease

CHAPTER 30

1. Refer to Chapter 30 for a complete description.
2. Final impression, die construction
3. Refer to Chapter 30 for a complete description.

4. Refer to Chapter 30 for a complete description.
5. Refer to Chapter 30 for a complete description.
6. Refer to Chapter 30 for a complete description.
7. f
8. c
9. g
10. d
11. a
12. b
13. e
14. b
15. a
16. b
17. a
18. a
19. d
20. c

CHAPTER 31

1. Refer to Chapter 31 for a complete description.
2. Refer to Chapter 31 for a complete description.
3. Refer to Chapter 31 for a complete description.
4. f
5. g
6. d
7. b
8. j
9. h
10. a
11. c
12. c
13. c
14. c
15. T
16. T
17. T
18. F
19. F
20. F
21. T
22. F
23. F
24. T
25. F
26. T

CHAPTER 32

1. To prevent drifting, to provide esthetics, to protect tooth, to aid in mastication, to prevent hypereruption
2. a. Acrylic bridge
   b. Full coverage acrylic, polycarbonate crown

   c. Intracoronal temporary cement or acrylic
   d. Full coverage acrylic crown
   e. Full coverage metal/acrylic crown
3. d
4. d
5. c
6. c
7. b
8. a
9. b
10. d
11. d
12. d
13. c
14. d

CHAPTER 33

1 to 6. Refer to Chapter 33 for complete descriptions.
7. a
8. b
9. c
10. d
11. F
12. F
13. T
14. F
15. F
16. F
17. T
18. F
19. T

CHAPTER 34

1. a. TMJ surgery
   b. Trauma treatment
   c. Orthognathic
   d. Pathology
   e. Preprosthetic treatment
   f. cleft palate repair
2. a. Extractions
   b. Preprosthetic
   c. Biopsy
3. a. Do not rinse forcefully
   b. Do not use straws
   c. Keep pressure on site for 30 to 45 minutes
   d. Do not brush teeth in the area of the extraction for 24 to 48 hours
   e. Do not smoke for 24 hours
4. a. Pain
   b. Swelling
   c. Bleeding

d. Stiffness
e. Discoloration
5.
6. b
7. f
8. h
9. e
10. i
11. d
12. a
13. j
14. g
15. c
16. d
17. c
18. c
19. b
20. d

CHAPTER 35

1. Refer to Chapter 35 for a complete description.
2. Refer to Chapter 35 for a complete description.
3. Refer to Chapter 35 for a complete description.
4. a
5. d
6. d
7. a
8. b
9. d
10. b
11. b
12. d
13. a
14. b

CHAPTER 36

1. Refer to Chapter 36 for a complete description.'
2. Refer to Chapter 36 for a complete description.
3. Refer to Chapter 36 for a complete description.
4. d
5. c
6. F
7. T
8. F
9. F
10. F
11. F
12. F
13. F
14. F

CHAPTER 37

1. Refer to Chapter 37 for a complete description.
2. Refer to Chapter 37 for a complete description.
3. Refer to Chapter 37 for a complete description.
4. Refer to Chapter 37 for a complete description.
5. Refer to Chapter 37 for a complete description.
6. Refer to Chapter 37 for a complete description.
7. Refer to Chapter 37 for a complete description.
8. b
9. b
10. d
11. b
12. c
13. d
14. c
15. b
16. a
17. c
18. b
19. b
20. c
21. d

CHAPTER 38

1. Refer to Chapter 38 for a complete description.
2. Refer to Chapter 38 for a complete description.
3. Refer to Chapter 38 for a complete description.
4. Refer to Chapter 38 for a complete description.
5. Refer to Chapter 38 for a complete description.
6. Refer to Chapter 38 for a complete description.
7. b
8. d
9. F
10. T
11. F
12. T
13. T
14. T
15. T

CHAPTER 39

1. Any five of the following:
   Pouring impressions
   Trimming diagnostic models
   Constructing custom made trays
   Constructing baseplates
   Constructing mouthguards
   Constructing copings
   Creating waxed patterns for investment
   Casting metal restorations
2. Any eight of the following:

1. *No smoking* should be a general rule in the entire office. It is especially important not to smoke in the laboratory since many flammable agents are used in this area.
2. Safety glasses must be worn when operating any rotary equipment such as the dental lathe, model trimmer, or handpiece; when using the bunsen burner; or when chipping away plaster or stone from models.
3. Hair should be pulled back and secured. Long hair can become entangled in rotary devices. Bending over a bunsen burner can also be a potential hazard, if hair is not secured.
4. Hanging jewelry or clothing such as chains or scarves should not be worn. Like long hair, any dangling clothing simply enhances the chance for an accident.
5. Do not lean over a bunsen burner or a torch. Also, be certain to turn off these devices completely before leaving the area.
6. If a handpiece with an engine belt is used, change the belt frequently to avoid unexpected breaks in the belt. Maintain adequate tension on the belt to eliminate undue stress.
7. Keep electrical cords out of areas where water is used.
8. Turn off lathes, handpieces, model trimmers, or other rotary devices when not in use.
9. Use acceptable ventilation and exhaust systems when working with dental materials such as acrylic or when grinding on the lathe.
10. Follow OSHA guidelines for the handling of laboratory materials and substances.

3. Any 10 of the following:
1. Clean and disinfect work benches daily.
2. Disinfect work pans as soon as possible after removing an appliance, to make certain that they have been decontaminated before being used again.
3. Do not eat or drink at laboratory work stations.
4. Do not use the same pumice for new work and repair work. For repair work, premeasure pumice in small amounts and discard it after each use. Discard pumice that is used for new work weekly.
5. Wet pumice with a mixture of disinfectant and bacteriostatic soap. Do not use water alone.

6. Soak brush wheels and rag wheels in a disinfectant for 10 minutes, and allow to air dry overnight.
7. After using pumice on a repair, disinfect the appliance for 10 minutes. These materials are only surface disinfectants: when the material is cut or broken, the appliance must be disinfected again.
8. Use universal precautions, masks, glasses or face shield, and gloves when operating mechanical devices. Note: Use the dust-mist type of face masks in the laboratory. All face masks that are used in the dental laboratory should be NIOSH approved.
9. Use an effective suction or vacuum system when grinding an appliance.
10. Keep disinfectant solutions readily available in the laboratory.
11. In states where denturism is legal, the denturist is responsible for following the same infection control procedures that are used in the dental treatment room regarding contact with patient's secretions.

4. Any 10 of the following:
1. Product or chemical identity THAT IS used on the label
2. Manufacturer's or supplier's name and address
3. Chemical and common names of each hazardous ingredient
4. Name, address, and phone number for hazard and emergency information
5. Preparation or revision date of MSDS
6. The hazardous chemical's physical and chemical characteristics, such as vapor pressure and flash point
7. Physical hazards, including the potential for fire, explosion, and reactivity known health hazards
8. OSHA-permissible exposure limit (PEL), ACGIH threshold limit value (TLV), or other exposure limits
9. Emergency and first-aid procedures
10. Whether OSHA, NTP, or IARC lists the ingredient as a carcinogen
11. Precautions for safe handling and use
12. Control measures such as engineering controls, work practices, hygienic practices, or personal protective equipment required
13. Primary routes of entry
14. Procedure for spills, leaks, and clean-up

5. Review this question with your instructor or dentist to be certain that you have entered the correct data. For information on how to make this entry refer to Chapter 39 of the textbook.
6. d
7. a
8. e
9. c
10. h
11. g
12. T
13. T
14. F
15. F
16. T
17. F
18. T
19. F
20. F

CHAPTER 40

1. Anatomic, art
2. Curve of Spee
3. Any six of the following:
   1. Record the occlusal relationship of both dental arches in centric relation for present and future treatment
   2. Provide three-dimensional study of the relationship of the alveolar processes
   3. Allow study of tooth and occlusal relationships from the lingual aspect
   4. Allow study of tooth positioning, dental arch form, and occlusal relationships without the patient being present
   5. Act as teaching aids in case presentations and patient education
   6. Used to demonstrate changes that occur during and after treatment
   7. Provide reproduction of actual arch for use in constructing auxiliary devices such as custom-made trays or copings
   8. Function as legal records for insurance companies, malpractice suits, or forensic purposes
   9. Symmetrically trimmed models provide the opportunity to study asymmetries in the dental arches
4. Negative, positive
5. Any five of the following:
   1. All plaster and stone surfaces must be free of voids and bubbles.
   2. The union between the stone in the anatomic portion and the plaster base should be continuous and free of voids.
   3. The anatomic portion of the cast (dental arch and alveolar process) must be centered on the plaster base to provide adequate plaster on all sides for proper trimming.
   4. The occlusal plane of the dental arch should be parallel to the bottom of the rapid stone base.
   5. The base must be thick enough to provide adequate plaster for trimming the casts to the proper height.
   6. The anatomic portion of the cast must have sufficient vestibular and posterior extension to allow for proper depth of model trimming.
   7. The tongue area on the mandibular model should be free of excess plaster or stone.
6. Any 10 of the following:
   1. Backs of the models must be located posterior to the maxillary tuberosity and posterior to the most posterior mandibular tooth.
   2. Backs of the maxillary and mandibular models must be in the same plane.
   3. When articulated in occlusion, backs of the models should set flush on a flat surface without any movement of the occlusion.
   4. Base of the maxillary and mandibular models should be parallel to each other.
   5. All of the angles should be symmetric from side to side.
   6. All of the trimmed sides opposite each other should be the same height.
   7. Art portion of the maxillary model should be one third of the total height of the model.
   8. When articulated together, the models should be double the height of the maxillary model when the 2-maxillary occlusal plane is parallel to a flat surface.
   9. Occlusal plane should be at an angle between 0 to 5 degrees to the bases.
   10. Occlusal plane should be centered in the total height of the model.
   11. Midline of the maxillary model should be established at the posterior two thirds of maxillary palatal raphe.
   12. Flat cuts and angles should be symmetric with the midline.

13. Vertical cut lines should be parallel to each other and at a 90-degree angle to the base.

14. Sides should be trimmed to the greatest depth of the vestibule without destroying anatomical structure.

15. Models should be finished with smooth sides and bases; bubbles and voids removed or filled; sharp line angles; smooth tongue space

7. Missing teeth, severe malocclusion, an asymmetric arch

8. All five of the following:
   1. Accuracy in the impression is improved because there will be a better fit of the tray.
   2. An uniform thickness of the impression will be established between the tissues and tray walls to eliminate a potential for voids.
   3. Use of stops keeps the tray from resting on occlusal or incisal surfaces and consequently prevents "burn through" on dentulous trays.
   4. Less impression material required to fill the tray.
   5. Tray design can be altered to compensate for missing teeth, unusual arch form, tori, or small mouth openings.

9. Any 10 of the following:
   1. Free of voids or wrinkles
   2. Uniform thickness
   3. Smooth, even peripheral borders
   4. Free of lateral rocking
   5. Stops are well defined
   6. Dentulous tray extends 2 to 3 mm below the cervical border
   7. Border of edentulous tray extends to the greatest depth of the vestibule
   8. Full-arch tray extends posterior to the maxillary tuberosity or the retromolar pad
   9. A tray with full palatal coverage does not extend distal to the foveal area
   10. Handles are at least ½ inch but no more than ¾ inch in length and are at an angle to provide easy removal from the mouth
   11. Stops are marked on the exterior surface
   12. Interior surface is free of debris

10. Any five of the following:
   1. Close adaptation to anatomic structures
   2. Uniform thickness throughout
   3. Smooth, peripheral borders
   4. Extends to the maxillary tuberosity
   5. Should not impinge on vestibular or gingival tissue
   6. Should not impinge on frenii

11. c
12. b
13. a
14. a
15. a
16. a
17. a
18. b
19. d
20. b
21. c
22. d
23. T
24. F
25. T
26. F
27. T